Doing Health Anthropology: Research Methods for Community Assessment and Change

Christie W. Kiefer is Professor Emeritus of Anthropology in the Department of Anthropology, History, and Social Medicine in the School of Medicine, University of California, San Francisco. Over the past 20 years, Kiefer has done action research in Honduras, Nicaragua, Mexico, Ecuador, South Africa, Thailand, the Philippines, and Berkeley, California, working with medically underserved communities to improve their access to basic health services. He also teaches anthropology to medical and nursing students at UCSF, and serves on the board of directors of Lifelong Medical Care, a community-owned non-profit clinic in Berkeley, California. His writings include *Health Work with the Poor: A Practical Guide* (2000), *Refuge of the Honored: Social Organization in a Japanese Retirement Community* (1992), and *Changing Cultures, Changing Lives: An Ethnographic Study of Three Generations of Japanese Americans* (1974). Kiefer received his Ph.D. in cultural anthropology at the University of California, Berkeley, in 1968.

Doing Health Anthropology: Research Methods for Community Assessment and Change

Christie W. Kiefer, PhD

Professor of Anthropology, Emeritus
Department of Anthropology,
History, and Social Medicine
University of California—San Francisco

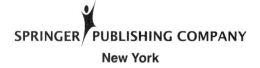

SPRINGER PUBLISHING COMPANY

New York

Springer Publishing Company, LLC
11 West 42nd Street
New York, NY 10036

Acquisitions Editor: *Jennifer Perillo*
Managing Editor: *Mary Ann McLaughlin*
Production Editor: *Maggie Meitzler*
Cover design: *Mimi Flow*
Composition: *Techbooks*

07 08 09 10/5 4 3 2 1

Library of Congress Cataloging-in-Publication Data

Kiefer, Christie W.
Doing health anthropology: research methods for community assessment and
change / Christie W. Kiefer.
    p. cm.
  Includes bibliographical references and index.
  ISBN 0-8261-1557-8 (hardback: alk. paper)
1. Medical anthropology—Research—Methodology.
  2. Public health—Anthropological aspects—Research—Methodology. I. Title.

GN296.K54 2006
306.4′6107—dc22

                                        2006028260

Printed in the United States of America by Bang Printing.

Contents

Acknowledgments

I thank all of my students and my host communities in California, Ecuador, the Philippines, Honduras, Japan, Mexico, Missouri, Nicaragua, South Africa, and Thailand for teaching me most of what is in this book. Major ideas and inspiration have also come from my great mentor, George DeVos, and from Jeremiah Mock, Daniel Perlman, Kira Foster, Suriya Wankankathep, Juan Almendares, and the late Masuda Kokichi. I also thank my editor at Springer Publishing Company, LCC, Jennifer Perillo, for many improvements to this book.

Preface

In recent years, as curative medicine has become both more effective and more expensive, it is clear that many people lack access to the best procedures. Accordingly, there has been a rapid increase in the number of scientists and training centers that have turned their attention from high-technology curative treatment to primary care, disease prevention, and health promotion as solutions to the problems of access to health. This book was inspired by that trend, and seeks to accelerate and refine it by helping health workers learn to use the powerful tools of anthropology to gain insight into the social causes of ill health.

This book offers one teacher's view of the basic ideas, attitudes, and skills that are needed by anyone who wants to do anthropological research on community health. It is the result of some 30 years of teaching anthropology to students in medicine, nursing, and public health – most of whom entered my classes with little or no background in the social sciences.

I have tried to write everything in direct, plain language, and to avoid social science jargon, so that anyone can follow my reasoning. However, cultural anthropology offers a way of looking at the world that is quite different from the ways of either the physical sciences or everyday consciousness. It takes some careful attention to really absorb this new way of seeing. This book has been written with cross-science communication as its constant theme. It is not a common theme in social science writing, and the language and point of view offered here may seem at first a bit strange to many. I can only say that experience has led me by many small steps to this way of presenting my subject.

Clear knowledge of the anthropological way of seeing ultimately comes from actually *doing* anthropology – experiencing personally the discovery of a pattern of human thought or activity of the sort anthropologists call *culture*. It is a little like playing chess or mah-jongg – the doing and the thinking are so interlinked. Ideally, then, this book should be read in group settings where the readers have an opportunity to practice what is being taught, and to help each other understand that experience.

The thirteen chapters that follow can be divided into four broad sections. Chapters One through Four explore the relationship between anthropological thought and method on one hand, and the concepts and methods of the physical sciences and medicine on the other hand. We begin by explaining why the leading concepts of health science need to be complemented with anthropological thinking. We then delve deeper into the hidden assumptions of the physical sciences, and show why these limit our ability to think creatively about human behavior. We explore the basic assumptions of an alternative philosophy – *the naturalistic theory of knowledge* – which informs anthropological thinking.

Chapters Five through Eight lay out a step-by-step path toward mastering the skills needed for doing anthropological research. By skills I mean not only procedures, but also ways of thinking about what one is doing and seeing, and ways of managing the human interactions that make up this kind of research. Health professionals especially should benefit from a deeper self-awareness of the way they relate to people in the communities they serve. I should also point out that the procedures I outline for recording and analyzing data need not be taken as final. There is wide room for individual choice in how to do these things, and there are plenty of books by highly skilled researchers that offer other ways. Every student needs to experiment with a variety of techniques, just as artists experiment with painting methods, to find those that are the most personally satisfying.

Chapters Nine and Ten are theoretical. They offer examples of useful ways of thinking about the main concerns of community health workers – the relationship of health to human nature and human needs, the impact of change and stress on communities, and the processes by which communities confront and overcome their own problems. Again, I make no claim that these theories are superior to the scores of others in the literature of the social sciences. I offer them as catalysts that can be used in the initial formation of research questions. In my view, good community health research draws from many theoretical sources, picking and choosing concepts that seem to make useful sense of the data.

Chapters Eleven, Twelve, and Thirteen go beyond basic research skills, adding abilities that are often useful for health scientists pursuing social problems. *Action anthropology*, in Chapter Eleven, is the term I apply to the role of the researcher as a direct participant and ally in helping communities improve their health. Teaching anthropological research methods to health workers who want to use them in their professions is another special skill, covered in Chapter Twelve. Finally, Chapter Thirteen addresses some of the issues raised by naturalistic research methods, and ways in which those issues have been addressed – including possible complementary approaches between naturalistic and laboratory research methods. I have included these chapters not merely as options, but because I also think they add a deeper perspective to the research enterprise itself. In other words, I think students as well as instructors might benefit from reading them, even if they do not plan to apply them directly in their work.

Aside from this preface, the reader of this book will find relatively few references to the abundant, excellent literature on the methods and philosophy of health social science. I arrived at the decision to write it this way through years of teaching anthropology to health scientists. This experience underlines what should be obvious to anyone at all familiar with both health science and social science – that the two areas have highly distinct traditions about what kinds of questions are important, how those questions should be answered, and what vocabularies and persuasive styles belong in scholarly writing. The vast majority of formal, published health social science studies – even those done by health practitioners – are written so as to satisfy the interests and meet the standards of social scientists of one kind or another. In many cases, this means that such studies are simply not useful to health practitioners, that is, they either address issues that are of little clinical or public health interest, or the issues are addressed in such a way that most practitioners lack the conceptual tools to fully understand the work's utility. While I certainly don't want to discourage health scientists from pursuing a professional level of social science training, I see my primary task in this book as that of making anthropological methods themselves directly accessible to as many health workers as possible. Besides, there are so many good books on methods for social scientists that yet another one that covers the same general ground in the same general way is hardly needed.

My great hope is that, as more and more health professionals recognize the need for the kinds of skills this book teaches, the ideas set forth here will be revised and refined by many hands. Perhaps the use of anthropological methods by skilled health professionals will one day become a broad and deep stream in the search for human betterment.

Doing Health Anthropology:
Research Methods for Community
Assessment and Change

CHAPTER ONE

Why Anthropology?

GUIDE TO THIS CHAPTER

This chapter describes the concept of *culture*, which is what distinguishes anthropological thinking and research. Culture is seen as a complex, integrated system of thought and behavior shared by members of a group – a system whose whole pattern allows us to understand the meanings that people attach to specific facts and observations. Because the cultural system is all-encompassing, and because most of it is not conscious at any particular time, anthropological research requires us to study a wide range of behaviors and situations in order to find the answer to any particular question. Because every sane human being thrives by understanding how his or her own cultural pattern works, we can use skills that we have already learned, in order to understand how other cultures work.

Next, we discuss the advantages of using this anthropological perspective in order to understand health and illness. The dominant model for understanding health is the *disease model*, which focuses on biological processes, and on the behaviors that directly produce these. However, there is wide agreement that a highly efficient way of promoting health is to promote healthy behavior. We examine why this is a process that is difficult to understand using the disease model, or even using the model of knowledge that most health researchers use. By allowing us to understand *why* people live as they do, anthropology opens the door to helping communities live in more healthy ways. This *why* question has many dimensions, including people's culture, environment, and economy, and how these things are changing over time.

WHAT IS CULTURAL ANTHROPOLOGY?
THE CONCEPT OF CULTURE

Like the other branches of social science (sociology, psychology, political science, and economics), anthropology developed mainly in Europe and

North America in the nineteenth century. At the time, scholars from this part of the world were just discovering the great diversity of human life and behavior. Many felt that a science was needed to make sure that the quickly growing store of knowledge about all the world's people could be recorded, taught, and made systematic. In short, anthropology is the study of the whole human species in all its diversity. Although this includes human social and physical evolution, human genetics, languages, arts, and many other sub-fields, in this book I am only concerned with one branch of anthropology, namely *cultural anthropology*, or the study of contemporary human cultures.

Cultural anthropology, then, is a social science that developed out of the discovery that every group of people who share a common history has certain highly patterned ways of thinking and behaving that members of the group share with each other, but not with the members of other groups who do not share their history. These patterns are called the group's *culture*. Cultural anthropology is the social science devoted to the study of human cultures. A culture is defined as the entire pattern of belief and behavior that is learned and shared by people as members of a social group. Important features of this definition are as follows:

1. Culture is a comparative concept. It directs attention to the shared, patterned similarities and differences between the behaviors of human groups. For example, suppose that most people in one society ("Society A") believe that disease is caused by microscopic organisms, and people in another society ("Society B") believe that disease is caused by witchcraft. Each of these two societies has ways of treating disease based on its dominant belief. This difference is called a *cultural* difference. If all the human groups in the world thought and behaved the same, there would be no need for the concept of culture.

2. Culture refers to behavior that is shared by members of a group. Within any human group, there are many ideas and behaviors that differ from person to person or family to family. Anthropologists build up their ideas about shared behavior by looking at similarities of individual thought and behavior within the group, and how these differ from the shared similarities of people in other groups. In an Islamic society, for example, there might be many different interpretations of the religion of Islam, but nearly everyone believes in basic Islamic concepts of right and wrong. In a Christian society, likewise, there are many ways of thinking about Christian values, but these are systematically different in some ways from basic Islamic values.

3. Culture is a holistic concept. Anthropologists think of a particular way of life as an integrated pattern of belief and behavior, the details of which fit together in a way that makes sense to the members of that culture. The job of the cultural anthropologist is not just to find out how the details of one group's culture differ from another's, but to show how these details add up to a coherent view of the world. If we take the example I just gave, of beliefs about the cause of disease, we will see that each belief is part of a general pattern of belief and behavior in each culture. People in Society A will have beliefs about where microscopic organisms come from, where they are found, how they affect the body, and how to prevent and get rid of the sickness they cause. They will recognize specialists whose job is to know about bacteria and viruses, and to deal with their effects. People in Society B will have theories about how different kinds of witchcraft work on the body, how to protect against it and treat it, and they too will recognize specialists in the art of diagnosing and treating the action of witches. Even more broadly, each one's belief about disease will make sense within the society's more general ideas about nature and the supernatural, about good and evil, about power, politics, economics, and fate.

4. As a result of this holistic view, each cultural system is considered unique. Every social group, even one as small as a village or a neighborhood, has its own individual history, and is a collection of individual personalities. We can talk about *national culture* when we compare how a typical Thai community today is different from a typical English one, or how the average American thinks differently from the average Japanese, but if we really want to understand the thinking of people in a village in any of these nations, we need to understand the unique experience and practices of that village, at this time in history.

5. Cultural behavior is not genetically inherited, it is learned by people as members of their society. If a genetically African child is brought up in a Chinese family, that child will learn Chinese culture, just as well as a genetically Chinese child would. Being learned, culture can be – and is – modified over the course of time. However, because its details form parts of a complex pattern, changes usually proceed slowly, and can cause severe psychological and social stress if they happen too fast, as we shall see later in this book.

6. Culture is a feature of all human life that has value in itself to the people who share it. Sharing beliefs and behaviors makes people

feel secure, gives meaning to their lives, and protects them from anxiety and confusion. Shared traditions are never emotionally neutral. They are things that people treasure and fight for, and if they are challenged in any way, the result is almost always suffering, and sometimes violence. This is a critical feature of culture and one that health workers must think about. Often, we believe that we need to change cultural habits in order to improve health. We need to realize that we are dealing with structures that are themselves important for sustaining health, and always act knowledgeably and with caution.

How Do Cultural Anthropologists Collect Data?

Cultural anthropology clearly overlaps with other social sciences, such as sociology and psychology, which are also often interested in human thought and behavior, and in the differences between social groups. What distinguishes anthropology from these other sciences is our focus on the comparative study of cultural systems as wholes. Sociologists might be interested in how different societies approach a particular problem, or produce a particular economic or political result; or they might be interested in particular aspects of a culture, such as social organization or religion. Psychologists might want to know how culturally unique ways of raising children produce certain personality traits in adults, or in how beliefs about health affect people's health related behavior. But only anthropologists focus their main attention on trying to understand the overall patterns that underlie the whole range of cultural thought and behavior – to understand the relationships among religion, science, economy, politics, art, health, technology, and history.

Because of this focus on interrelationships, on how the whole way of life fits together into a distinct whole, cultural anthropologists have an unusual way of working. This way of working is usually called *participant observation*. That means that, as much as possible, we try to live in the settings – villages, towns, dwellings, fields, forests, work places – where the people we are studying live and work. We try to do this for a year or more, so that we can see the entire cycle of daily, weekly, and seasonal change and observe all common events like births, rituals, illnesses, and deaths. And as much as possible, we try to participate in the normal everyday life of the people, so that we can directly observe as well as ask about what they do and how they think about it, and so that we can feel with our bodies and our senses what life in that culture is like.

The relationship between this method and the idea that culture is an integrated system should be clear. An integrated system is one in which each part is essential for the functioning of the whole. An example could be the human body. We cannot understand how humans are able to live unless we understand all parts of the body – how nutrition and oxygen are processed and distributed to the cells by all the organs, how the brain and nervous system regulate all these activities, how the sense organs allow us to regulate our behavior, how the muscles and bones work to sustain the system, and so on. Likewise in a culture, we cannot understand people's health related behavior unless we know their religious and scientific beliefs, the kinds of work they do, how they have adapted to their physical environment, what the possibilities of their technology are, what they believe about right and wrong, who wields power, how, and for what purposes, and how this has all evolved through a specific historical process that left its mark on people's experience and belief.

Since this book is written for health workers, and since health workers might not be able to use the methods of cultural anthropology in their ideal form, we will discuss ways that these methods can be adapted to different work situations.

How Do Cultural Anthropologists Analyze Data?

Another very important feature of cultural anthropology that makes it somewhat different from other sciences is the way we analyze data. Our overall strategy may use statistical data and even survey results, but in the end it is qualitative and descriptive. Again beginning with the proposition that cultures are unique, integrated wholes, anthropologists do not assume that the relationship between *facts* (measurements, observations, or verbal reports) can be understood, without viewing those *facts* in operation, in the context of the whole system of living and belief. The main analytic activity in cultural anthropology is the search for pattern. In order to identify patterns, anthropologists sometimes list measurements in tables and look for statistical correlations between variables, but that is never enough. If such measurements seem to indicate a pattern, the anthropologist wants to use direct observation to find out what other cultural regularities are related to this pattern – in other words to see how a simple relationship is part of the complex whole, or even whether the correlation is merely accidental or uninteresting. Only when this is clear can the analysis be called anthropological.

For this reason, in anthropology, analysis and data collection proceed together, from the first day of the study to the last. The meaning of an observation, and its bearing on the purpose of the study, cannot be taken for granted. It must be tested whenever possible. Each observation leads to many new questions. Is this behavior typical, or unusual? What does it mean to the people who do it? How is it related to their other beliefs and behaviors? What are the alternatives in this culture (if any)? If two behaviors look similar, do they mean the same thing for the actors? How does the context of a behavior change its meaning? In this book, we will discuss many of the ways anthropologists seek the underlying patterns that make sense out of measurements and observations.

I'm afraid I have made anthropology sound like very, very hard work. Actually, it is easy and fun once you understand the basic idea. Anthropology uses the same skills all of us have used all our lives, naturally, without even thinking about them, as we learn to live in our own culture. Every day, you are using your skills of pattern recognition when you understand what people say, appreciate a work of art, recognize a familiar person or place, make a judgment about what to buy, detect an error in your work, or realize that someone likes you. Anthropology consists mostly of making such skills conscious and perfecting them, so that you become more accurate, more confident, and more persuasive in your understanding of human behavior. By the way, this makes anthropology very useful in your private life as well.

THE ADVANTAGES OF ANTHROPOLOGY FOR THE HEALTH SCIENCES

It is now widely accepted in public health that preventing illness and promoting good health are cost effective ways of improving the health of populations and avoiding some of the health threats that become more serious as societies become more modern and affluent. Of course, health promotion and disease prevention involve changing the way people think and behave. In order to do this, it is important to know the ways in which people are now thinking and acting that may affect their health, and what kinds of new actions will make sense to them and help them accept changes.

Also, it is widely accepted that some of the new attitudes and ways of life that are spreading rapidly around the world as a result of faster communication and transportation have the possibility of endangering healthy local practices. New technology, leisure, and wealth also carry an element of danger. Anthropology offers a powerful, systematic way of understanding what factors are affecting people's health, and how to evaluate public health plans that affect people's behavior.

To understand how anthropology can improve on the models of behavior that are now most widely used in the health sciences, let us look closely at these existing models.

The Mighty Disease Model

The modern health sciences, including human and animal medicine, pharmacy, and to a large extent also nursing and public health, are based on a model of knowledge often called the *disease model*. This model uses the powers of laboratory science and statistics to gain detailed and precise knowledge of how bodies function and how physical diseases work. Statistics are used to study natural settings such as clinics and communities. The public health method of studying human behavior is based on the same assumptions as the laboratory study of disease, as we will discuss in a moment.

The great success of laboratory science derives from its five-step method:

1. one develops precise models of cause and effect based on everything that is known about a problem;
2. one predicts how each small isolated variable of each model will behave under carefully controlled conditions;
3. one creates those conditions and measures how the isolated variables behave;
4. one refines the models to take account of unpredicted variation; and
5. one repeats this process with each new variable of each new model until the predicted results are seen; or until one can explain, using accepted theory, why they are not seen.

Using the disease model based on such laboratory-like studies, scientists can craft ingenious ways to discover subtle causes of illness in the body. They can isolate a specific bacterium, virus, genetic defect, or injury that causes a specific illness; and they can often discover ways to control the infection or defect, or repair the damage it has done. They can continuously improve treatment and care procedures so that health workers can improve the healing effects of their work on the bodies of patients. They can devise ways for people to live and work that lower the risk of illness and promote long, healthy lives. There is nothing surprising about the fact that the laboratory- and statistics-based disease model plays such an important role in the health sciences.

But the disease model is limited in what it can do to improve health. It needs to be used together with other models that address equally important health problems that cannot be studied properly using traditional laboratory techniques. These other problems arise from all the life processes related to health that are highly complex, unstable, and unpredictable.

Much of health-related behavior is easily disrupted by our efforts to study it in a laboratory-like model, because people behave differently when they are being controlled and measured. It is hard to understand how a behavior is related to an illness if there are many events and steps involved in the connection.

For example, in many places illnesses are treated by a combination of meditation, prayer, ritual, and physical touch. If one tries to find out whether these techniques work, using a laboratory science model of study, think about what happens:

1. First, every step in the procedure must be studied separately, to see which, if any, of the steps is having an effect. This of course completely changes the process of the cure if it is ordinarily performed the same way each time, without interruption between steps.
2. Second, the state of the patient must be carefully measured both before and after the treatment. If patients' conditions are too different at the beginning, the results will not be valid. But the process of measuring their states amounts to a whole new element in the ritual of healing, and might completely change the results.
3. Third, the outcome of the cure might depend on some subtle qualities of the relationship between the patient and the healers. If an unknown person – the researcher – enters into the healing process, this relationship might be changed in such a way that the results are different.
4. Many other possible distortions of the natural process might also be taking place. The experiment might have to be done in an artificially controlled environment, and so on.

In other words, many behaviors cannot be broken down into measurable variables that can be managed and exactly measured by the researcher. They are affected by all of the social, cultural, economic, environmental, historical, and political processes that shape how people live, think, work, interact, and maintain or lose their health. Let us refer to all the ways of approaching these other problems collectively as the *social perspective* on health and health care.

The Social Perspective on Health

The social perspective is much harder to describe than the disease model. Its basic idea is to look at the health of individuals and groups not simply as the result of carefully measured factors such as bacteria, or blood cortisol levels, or genetic traits, or even measurable behaviors like smoking or sugar intake. Rather, the social perspective tries to understand the whole environment of the person or group as a complex, interacting system that produces health outcomes through multiple pathways. It often uses exact measurements, such as rates of a particular disease or behavior, but it uses them as indicators of more complex processes that cannot be accurately measured.

Let us return to the example of naturalistic healing I just gave: Using the social perspective, a researcher would try to observe many cases of the healing process just the way it is ordinarily carried out. Careful notes would record just what was done each time, and what happened to the patient afterward. The researcher would try to observe people with similar symptoms who were treated in different ways or by different healers, to see what observations seemed to go together. Moreover, the researcher would be interested not just in the physical effects of the treatment, but also in its effects on the rest of the patient's life, and the life of his community and family. An attempt would be made to understand how different ways of treating certain symptoms fit into the complex pattern of life of the community.

Another good example of the social perspective is the attempt to understand why people in some societies live longer than in others. In England during the latter nineteenth century, life expectancy began to climb dramatically, and birth rates began to fall, *before* the disease model had even discovered most diseases, let alone devised vaccines and treatments to prevent or cure them. A thorough study of everything that was happening in English society at that time shows that many more people gained access to a nutritious diet, that housing and sanitation began to improve, and – perhaps most important of all – millions of people began to feel more hopeful about their futures and their children's future than their parents had. This discovery is not very surprising to us any more, but if we examine the details of it, it has a great deal of power in explaining health in the modern world, and in suggesting actions that will improve health.

Why Isn't the Social Perspective More Widely Used?

Nothing I have said so far is new. Scholars have recognized the social and economic causes of illness for more than 150 years, and the limitations of the disease model were discussed in medical journals almost as soon as that model itself appeared in the late nineteenth century. Why, then, must I restate these often-repeated truths? Why is the disease model so one-sidedly triumphant over the social perspective? There are six interrelated reasons:

1. The disease model has been brilliantly successful in reducing suffering and death from disease in most of the world. It has also succeeded in a more dramatic way than the advances in nutrition and sanitation that contributed even more to world health at the same time. In the public mind, it is the curative medicine of the disease model, not the health improvements of the social perspective, that have led to our most important advances against sickness.
2. The social perspective rarely produces universal answers to problems. It seeks to understand health as a feature of its rich, complex, social surroundings. Those surroundings vary greatly from culture to culture, from era to era, and even from community to community. Accordingly, the findings of the social perspective approach are usually limited to certain situations, and each distinct situation must be studied anew. This does not mean, however, that the social perspective does not produce models and theories that can be used very effectively over and over. Once a *fit* has been established between the models developed in one situation and the conditions of another situation, social models can be highly efficient.
3. The solution to one community's problems might not be applicable in another community, and "one size fits all" procedures often simply do not work. In addition, it takes considerable time to understand a community as a health system. In our fast-paced era, decision makers usually want answers quickly.
4. In many countries, especially the United States, the disease model has produced a health care industry that is extremely profitable for private investors. This is far less true of the social perspective. People – governments and charities as well as individuals – are simply willing to spend huge sums to cure disease, but reluctant to spend such sums on the more complicated tasks of avoiding it. The disease model, directed mainly at the physical effects of disease, lends itself to the development of marketable products such as drugs, medical equipment and supplies, research results, and measurable technical skills – things that can be produced and sold for a profit in a market economy.
5. The social perspective on health care has powerful political implications. It draws attention to those social practices and cultural attitudes that lead to poverty and social inequality, dangerous working and living conditions, poor environmental practices, and the marketing of unhealthy products, attitudes, and pastimes. It often draws attention to poor government, corruption, profiteering,

and discrimination against minorities, women, and the poor. As such, it disturbs powerful interests that profit from these features of society.

6. The disease model is based, as I mentioned, on a model of knowledge derived from the laboratory sciences, which occupy a powerful place in the belief and education systems of the urban industrial countries. The theory of knowledge needed to solve the non-biological, social-economic-political problems of health – I call it the naturalistic theory of knowledge – is radically different from that of the laboratory sciences. This naturalistic theory is not taught (nor is philosophy in general) in mainstream basic education, and is unfamiliar to all but the very few – to students of philosophy, in fact. My hardest task in this book will be to teach the basics of the naturalistic theory of knowledge.

The Advantages of the Social Perspective

In this book I do not elaborate on these reasons for health science's one-sided reliance on the disease model. I mention them only to help explain the need for an alternative. Later, I will discuss how the health professions have developed their own culture, and how this culture helps to stabilize and support the disease model. Now let us look more closely at the advantages of the social perspective, as understood through the study of anthropology. Let us consider the following:

1. Many causes of health and illness can only be understood from the study of the social, cultural, and historical surroundings of the people under study.
2. Such surroundings are extremely variable from place to place and time period to time period. Health promotion and illness prevention must be tailored to their actual, ongoing, local context.
3. Anthropology provides the tools for developing both this broader theoretical understanding, and this local, practical one.

   It is well known that certain social factors, like income, education, language, occupation, gender, and race, are strongly related to rates of illness in almost all societies. Some of the reasons for this appear obvious: People who cannot afford good housing in clean surroundings, safe jobs, adequate rest, good food and clothing, and medicine will suffer poorer health. People who have little knowledge of the actual causes of illness, or who believe in unsafe health practices, will be at greater risk of getting ill than those who have a lot of knowledge. People who are routinely the victims of deliberate violence or neglect will have greater health problems. Yet these are only a few of a large variety of ways social, cultural, and historical contexts affect health.

EXAMPLE: *Understanding and Treating Hypertension from a Social Perspective*

Hypertension is an illness that inflicts a huge burden of suffering and death, and if affects poor people far more than the middle class. It would be easy to assume that poor people suffer more stress than middle class people, and nothing can be done about this, but this produces no solution to the problem, and may not be accurate anyway. The risk of hypertension can be reduced by diet, exercise, medication, and stress reduction techniques, all things that are easier to manage for people who have money than those who do not. How can we design programs that public health departments can afford, and that improve the ability of poor people to reduce their blood pressure? The answer will vary tremendously according to how the hypertensive people in a particular neighborhood or cultural group live, and what usable resources are at hand. The answer, then, requires us to know both a great deal about the interactions of culture, income, diet, exercise, and stress, and how these interactions are expressed in a particular community.

A health worker equipped with anthropological methods will be able, if given enough time to observe life in the affected neighborhoods and talk with both hypertensive and normal people who live there, to answer many of these questions. He will observe what people eat and drink, what they do for leisure, how they work. He will learn from them what they like about certain foods and pastimes, and why they have the jobs they do. He will observe what their typical stresses and worries are, and what strategies they use to deal with these. He will also talk with employers, community leaders, merchants, and elected officials to understand what they think about the problem. He will develop an idea of the resources in the neighborhood that might be used to improve cardiac health. With this information in hand, he will be in a far better position than one trained in the disease model to assess what kinds of community health programs might reduce hypertension in this neighborhood.

4. The way people understand and deal with their own health and illness has a major effect on the kinds of health care they need. Anthropology offers tools for learning people's health related perceptions.

EXAMPLE: *Overcoming Cultural Barriers to Prenatal Care*

In my city, as in some others, babies of low-income African American women are much more likely than other babies to be underdeveloped at birth, and to suffer health problems as a result. This outcome is related to, among other things, a lack of prenatal care of the mothers. There are excellent prenatal care services available at no cost to the mothers, and almost all the mothers know about these services, but many do not use them. Why, and what can be done to correct this? The answer is not simply knowledge, or lack of access, or poverty, or even a combination of these things. The answer has to do with the entire way the women in this city live, what they value and want, and the experiences they have had with health care all their lives. Many of them feel unworthy of good care, and/or ambivalent about being pregnant, and/or mistrustful of the health care system, and/or fearful of the justice system and authority in general. To design a care system that will help them overcome these barriers will require a thorough knowledge both of the dynamics of racism and poverty in America, and of the specific details of local African American working class perceptions about their health, the health care system, and community resources.

With anthropological skills and the chance to use them, a health worker in this community will be able to identify women who need, but do not use, perinatal services. She will learn how they live; what they think about their health and health care; whom they trust and do not trust and why; how they understand their pregnancies and the health of their babies; and what kinds of help make them feel most comfortable. This information, in the hands of the perinatal care service providers, may lead to some ideas that will greatly improve pregnancy outcomes for women at risk.

5. Modern technology is changing social life at a faster and faster pace. This rapid change itself puts social and cultural systems under extreme strain, and produces serious health problems. Anthropology offers a way to understand social change.

EXAMPLE: Social Change and Illness in Rural Thailand

Right now, rural Thailand is experiencing an epidemic of amphetamine and alcohol use, and related problems of overdose, traffic accidents, violent crime, and sexually transmitted diseases, among teenagers. Why, and what can be done? To understand this problem, one must have a broad knowledge of the traditional culture, environment, and technology of rural Thailand, and of the massive and sudden changes that have arrived there in the last decade or two. A generation ago, there were few paved roads or motor vehicles, and most travel was done on foot or by small boat. Cash employment was very hard to find; there were few televisions, no cell phones or computers, and entertainment consisted mostly of festivals and celebrations that brought people of all generations and social classes together. Fashions and fads were beyond most young people's reach, even if they knew about them. Under the circumstances, surveillance and discipline of the young by families was rather relaxed and simple.

Suddenly, in the last decades, the picture is exactly the opposite. Motorbikes and paved roads make travel fast and easy for teenagers, and many commute to cash jobs away from home. Many have cell phone and e-mail contacts with others their age over a wide area. The kids watch MTV and hang out in malls stocked with every available novelty in clothes, music, and gadgetry. Mobility, cash, a hunger for the latest styles, and easy communication have helped produce a rebellion among teenagers that the parents have no way of understanding or coping with. (And this process is repeated in one way or another in "developing" cultures all over the world.)

Meanwhile, the growth of manufacturing in the countryside has pushed up land prices and brought in poorly paid migrant laborers who are exploited by local landlords and merchants, as well as by their employers. Some farmers sell or rent their land for huge profits and invest the proceeds in the new economy; and others are forced to sell their labor cheaply in a diluted market. New class divisions arise, so that some newly wealthy people become addicted to new fads and styles, and others suffer greatly from increased poverty and discrimination. Drug and alcohol abuse, violence, accidents, mental illness, and infectious disease have to be understood in this context.

What changes in education, law and enforcement, economic policy, and health care might help parents and children, laborers and health workers to address and solve this problem? Again, the answers require *both* an understanding of the broad social-historical stage on which the problem plays out, *and* an understanding of its specific dynamics in each rural community.

By researching written records and the memories of the local people, a health worker with anthropological training will be able to reconstruct the recent historical processes that are affecting health in their region, and how these processes have affected their own community. Trends, activities, and institutions that threaten local social life, and those that enhance it, can be more clearly identified. The indirect effects of new policies and interventions on the health of the community can be more clearly seen.

6. The health care professions are also unique cultural systems. As health care is an interaction between professional and local cultures, it is important to understand the professional side of the relationship as well.

We have already discussed how the popularity of the disease model of health care often blinds health workers to the need for a social perspective. There are many other unconscious assumptions that health professionals learn along with their professional skills, that strongly affect the way they relate to their clients, view their colleagues, and do their jobs. These assumptions can have great effects on health outcomes.

Perhaps the most important assumption of most health professional cultures is the way they think about the relationship between the caregiver and the patient. Of course health workers realize that individual patients react differently in similar situations, and that some health professionals are more skilled than others in building good relationships with patients. But there is a standard or ideal relationship that guides the way nearly all providers view and relate to patients – a model implied by the word *provider*, that we often use to describe the relationship. In this model, the relationship is an implied or explicit contract, in which there are three critical factors:

1. The *patient* (or his guardian) is an individual who seeks relief or protection from the provider. This signals that the patient or guardian
   (a) wants an illness to be cured or to be protected from an illness;
   (b) trusts the provider's superior knowledge and ability to help; and,
   (c) wants to answer the provider's questions and follow the provider's advice as well possible.
   The patient (or his guardian), then, alternates among the roles of:
   (a) client or petitioner, requesting a service;
   (b) experimental subject, providing data;
   (c) student, learning the action needed for the cure; and,
   (d) helper, carrying out the provider's instructions.
      If there is any doubt that he is really sick, or really wants to be treated, he deviates from the petitioner role. If he will not answer questions honestly, or allow himself to be examined and tested, he deviates from the subject role. If he does not listen to and remember, or believe, the provider's advice, he deviates from the student role. And if he does not carry out the provider's instructions, he deviates from the helper role. Any serious deviation in any role puts the contract under question. In the case of avoiding sickness, the patient roles still apply.
2. The *sickness* (or injury) is a physical problem, a disease, the antithesis of health. Health is always assumed to be the good, normal state of the body, and sickness always the result of a bad external agent or event that compromises this normal state. The role of sickness in the relationship can be understood clearly from the vocabulary used in the relationship. The patient and provider fight the sickness, which invades or attacks the body, by relying on the body's defenses, and the weapons of healing. The symptoms of sickness might include, or begin with, the patient's emotional and mental state, but if they have no measurable physical expression, the sickness is not "real," in which case the patient may be referred for psychiatric therapy, or the contract may be in question.

3. The *provider* knows, or should know, how to discover the physical cause of the sickness, and (except with incurable or chronic diseases) how to cure it. If this is not the case, the provider is obligated to say so, and to try to connect the patient with another provider who has the necessary knowledge and skill, if any. The provider first plays the role of
   (a) scientist, judge, and examiner. As soon as possible, the examiner must determine if the sickness or vulnerability is "real," and what might cause or prevent it. Later, the examiner determines the state or stage of the illness or healing;
   (b) teacher, explaining to the patient what must be done;
   (c) healer, actively treating the illness.

Note that the patient roles of petitioner, experimental subject, student, and helper, are passive or subordinate; and those of judge/examiner, teacher, and healer are active or dominant. Rarely, if ever, are these roles reversed.

In cultures where Western biomedicine is dominant, patients as well as providers are generally comfortable with this model of the relationship. However, as any good provider knows, the real relationship often does not match the model, and the result might be something unexpected. There are thousands of examples. The patient (let's say she is a woman) might complain about one set of symptoms, but might actually want help for something else, such as an emotional crisis; or she might not want any help at all, but instead might just be hoping to please a relative by going to the provider. Her view of what the sickness is might be completely different from the provider's, and she might be confused by what he says. She might not trust the provider at all, and might not have any intention to follow the advice she is given. She might have forgotten important things about the illness, or she might assume incorrectly that the provider knows things about her life that affect her health. She might not be able to do the things she is instructed, because they cost too much, or someone interferes, or because such things are not done in her tradition. She might decide to follow completely different advice given to her by someone else.

The provider (let's say he's a man) might not understand what the patient is saying, or might not believe her. He might not have the knowledge needed to understand her illness, or he might ask the wrong questions. If he knows very little about her life or culture (which is often the case), he might assume that she can understand or do things that she cannot, and so on.

A provider who understands his own assumptions as well as the patient's, and knows the ways in which those assumptions might be wrong, is in a much better position to avoid mistakes than one who does not. Anthropology gives a provider tools for understanding what assumptions he is making, and testing whether those assumptions will work in any given situation.

SUMMARY

Anthropology provides health professionals with a set of tools for understanding health and illness according to the social perspective. This perspective is important, because it makes clear the important relationships among health and culture, environment, economics, history, and individual thought and action. The usefulness of the social perspective has been known for over a hundred years, but it is not used as much as it should be. This is because health institutions in most modern societies have come to rely heavily on the disease model. The way of thinking about health according to the disease model is fundamentally different from the social perspective, although the two are not incompatible.

Anthropology teaches us how to think about human lives and communities as complex systems of which health is just one integral part. It teaches us how to understand the unspoken assumptions, feelings, logic, and communication habits that people use in everyday life and in health practice. It teaches us how to look at communities as products of a process of historical change. It gives us tools for examining our own assumptions about interactions, and how those assumptions affect outcomes.

In order to understand how anthropology does these things, it is first important to realize that the idea of *what constitutes knowledge* in anthropology differs from the ideas used by the disease model and its related sciences. Most health professionals were taught to think of knowledge according to ideas on which the disease model is based, and therefore we must learn how to recognize those ideas and put them aside, in order to use anthropology effectively. In the next chapter, we will compare these two theories of knowledge, and explain why the anthropological model is necessary for the social perspective on health.

CHAPTER TWO

Positivism: The Laboratory Theory of Knowledge

GUIDE TO THIS CHAPTER

In this chapter, we look closely at the ideas of *knowledge, truth*, and *validity*, the way these ideas are presented in the laboratory sciences, and in those types of social science that are based on the laboratory sciences, such as survey research. I want to emphasize at the beginning that nearly all social science, including the kind of cultural anthropology explained in this book, uses a blend of what I am calling laboratory-type methods and the naturalistic ones I will describe in the next chapter.

Very simply, the laboratory method allows scientists to study things in the most carefully controlled and well-documented way possible. Every step of the study procedure is described in detail, and the important features of it are measured to the finest degree.

This control and documentation allows other scientists to repeat the experience almost exactly, in order to ensure that the results that the original study produced were the correct ones (or not) – that is, whether the conclusions are *true*, and *valid*.

This way of working is based on three simple ideas:

(1) Everything in the universe can be reduced to basic laws, such as the laws of physics, and these laws are true always and everywhere, forever.
(2) We can learn these laws by eliminating the error of human judgment from our observations.
(3) We eliminate error by reducing our observations to simple procedures where we exactly measure and describe what happened, so that others can do and observe the same things.

THE MEANINGS OF *KNOWLEDGE*

The idea of *knowledge* is an abstraction, and like all abstractions, its actual meaning grows out of the use that groups of people make of it.

Every culture has its own way of thinking about what knowledge is. In Western cultures, it is a very complicated word that can mean many different things, depending on what we are talking about. In English, for example, we can say we "know that person," meaning we have seen him or know some facts about him. The same can be said about knowledge of any specific thing, like a place or an event, or a work of art, literature, or music. We can speak of this kind of knowledge as *experience*. It is made up mostly of memories stored in our brains, memories that we refresh and modify in our conversations with people.

A second way we say we know something is by listening to people explain things, and forming an opinion of who has understood them correctly. Here, we may not have any direct experience of the thing in question, but we use our beliefs about what is reasonable to form an *opinion*. Ideas about the value of people and things are typically formed this way. I might change my opinions, in which case, I have to admit I didn't really *know* what I thought I knew to begin with. However, opinions are usually the only kind of knowledge we have of that huge category of things we have not actually experienced, and we routinely behave as if our opinions were reliable knowledge.

A third way of knowing is meant when we say, "I know how to ride a bicycle," or "how to play tennis," or "how to read music." Here, we are talking about having mastered a skill, and the knowledge might not have any representation in our minds, other than the thought of doing the thing. The knowledge actually consists of automatic movements of our eyes and bodies. We can call this knowledge *practice*. Again, we can decide that we are doing something incorrectly, and change our knowledge of how to do it, but this does not mean we had no knowledge of it to begin with, only that our knowledge was faulty.

Then there is there is knowledge of a purely intellectual nature, which might be represented by things or events, but stands on its own, independent of them. Thus, how to tell the difference between truth and falsehood, or good and evil, or beauty and ugliness, is a kind of knowledge that tries to minimize the error that emotion and point of view introduce into knowing. We call this *theory*, or *philosophy*. Knowledge about truth is called *epistemology*, or the *theory of knowledge*; knowledge about goodness or justice is called *ethics*; and knowledge about beauty is called *aesthetics*.

Anthropology differs from the laboratory style of science that underlies the disease model as a form of knowledge in many ways. The two approaches often focus on different facts, for example, with disease theorists looking for statistical relationships between certain symptoms and the presence of certain specific microbes or bodily states, and anthropologists looking for patterns in the way belief and behavior seem to promote, or damage, wellness. They require different skills; in the one case laboratory technique and statistical calculation, and in the other case how to read a social situation and figure out how the actors themselves might understand the interaction. But we will get to those sorts of differences later in this book. For now, I want to focus on the different theories of knowledge used in the two ways of knowing.

POSITIVISM: THE LABORATORY SCIENCE
THEORY OF KNOWLEDGE

In real life, all scientific exploration actually uses a mixture of different theories of knowledge, but in laboratory science there is one theory that is usually dominant, and we call this theory *positivism*. Many books have been written about positivism, but in its simplest form, this theory proposes that:

- we live in a real universe that exists independently of our knowledge;
- this universe is not random, but adheres to eternally fixed principles, or regularities – it is predictable;
- we can gain knowledge of these regularities by studying the universe with our senses and using logic to infer how it works;
- we can distinguish between true and false knowledge;
- true knowledge is achieved by agreement among independent, trained observers making highly accurate observations of the same kinds of things; and
- statements about universal principles can be verified (proven true) by making predictions, then observing whether the predictions are always exactly fulfilled.

According to positivist theory, the *experimental method* is the best way to gain true knowledge. The experimental method is essentially a method by which:

- we develop precise models of cause and effect based on everything that is known about a question;
- we predict how each small isolated variable of each model will behave under carefully controlled conditions;
- we create those conditions and measure how the isolated variables behave;
- we refine the models to take account of unpredicted variation; and

- we repeat this process with each new variable of each new model until the predicted results are seen; or until one can explain, using accepted theory, why they are not seen.

Validity

The reason the experimental method is so useful, is that it divides natural processes into very small, simple parts. These parts can be described and measured exactly, and they can be subjected to procedures that can be described and re-created quite accurately by different experimenters at different times and places. The results of these procedures can also be accurately described and measured. If these exact procedures, followed by independent, trained observers, produce results that the experts agree are the same, we can say that "the experimental findings are confirmed." Note, then, that the criterion of validity in positivism is agreement among trained observers. Controlled experiments, which can be repeated in nearly exact detail by independent experimenters, are the gold standard for achieving this kind of agreement. Note also that a good deal of social science strives to imitate the replicability of experiments, for example by creating questionnaires and drawing random samples – things that can be done in much the same way by different researchers at different times and places.

Elegance and Parsimony

The next step in positivist science, of course, is to explain the findings. Here, sets of logical rules are used to select the best explanation. The two main signs of a good explanation are (1) *elegance*, that this particular explanation explains the largest possible number of findings, not just the single finding in question; and (2) *parsimony*, that this particular explanation is the simplest one that fits all the relevant observations, and fits most easily with all other relevant accepted explanations.

For example, take the theory that tuberculosis is caused by a bacterial infection. It is observed by independent trained observers that whenever a person has a specific set of observed symptoms, including a certain describable type of lesion in the lungs, you can look at tissue from these lesions under a microscope, and you with find bacilli that look a certain way. This theory has elegance and parsimony because: (1) it does not propose that some cases of these particular lesions are caused by one thing, and some cases caused by another; (2) it fits with observations of many other kinds of diseases, where one finds a particular kind of bacteria associated with a particular kind of lesion; (3) it also explains the fact that we can make someone sick with TB by exposing them to the bacteria; (4) it is in accord with the discovery that we can prevent the disease by reducing exposure to the bacteria, or strengthening the body's natural ability to fight off the infection; and, (5) it is in accord with a much wider body of theory that explains how microparasites infect human bodies, how the body fights these infections, and so on.

As I have said earlier, positivism is extremely powerful as a theory of knowledge because it allows us to construct theories that can be used in all sorts of practical ways, from curing disease to building global satellite television and phone systems. Later in this book, I will talk more about how the positivist theory of knowledge has influenced the way health scientists think about, and do, research, and why it leads to so many mistakes.

EXAMPLE: Ban Chan Village: Positivist versus Naturalistic Methods

A group of nurses had been working in a rural village we will call Ban Chan. The village had many health problems related to behavior (such as hypertension and accidents), and the nurses had not been very successful in getting the villagers to change the behaviors they thought were causing the problems. They decided to adopt social science methods to develop a different kind of project. In their understanding, the public health model they had been using in the past did not work because the authorities, not the villagers, had decided what to do. As a result, usually they could not get the cooperation of the people, who did not understand the public health concepts, or trust the authorities who were trying to change their lives.

Quite reasonably, the nurses did an opinion survey, asking the villagers what they thought the biggest problems in the village were. Two problems were mentioned more than any others: One was that people were fighting over the money controlled by the village council for business projects. The other was that the young people were throwing wild parties in places where the adults could not bother them, where they drank alcohol, had sex, and got into fistfights.

Because the villagers said these were important, the nurses reported that these two issues should be the top priorities for a public health project in the village. Their logic seemed clear: The villagers felt that these problems were causing too much stress, and wanted to be rid of them. They would be likely to cooperate with the health authorities, the project would be successful, and a good relationship would be established between the nurses and the villagers. They could then move on to other problems that the villagers also wanted solved.

The nurses' idea was intelligent from a laboratory science point of view. They constructed a model [people will cooperate if they feel their needs are being addressed], designed a method for assessing the key variables [what do they feel are their needs?] collected the data [opinion questionnaires], analyzed it [ranked the people's answers], and used it to set their own priorities.

Although intelligent, this plan did not work well. It was still hard to get the people to cooperate with the nurses, and the village continued to have these problems. The nurses decided they needed a different way of thinking, so they took a course in anthropology. They learned to think of social change as a process that involves the entire local culture, including the relationship between the villagers and the health care system.

Using their anthropological training, the nurses reevaluated their first attempt to design a project in Ban Chan. They realized they had overlooked several problems with it. First, their original model isolated a single "variable" [what do people think the worst problems are?] from its social context. Now, they realized that they needed to take part in village life, in order to find out why people think these problems are so important. They needed to seek in everyday conversation and activity the underlying dynamics of social organization, values, and social change that the problems implied. When, and only when, these dynamics were clear could they ask the question of whether, where, and how, to intervene.

Second, the original study did not address the basic nature and history of the relationship between the researchers as health experts, and the villagers as their clients. The researchers had not joined as equal participants in village life, so that they could contribute their knowledge naturally when and where the need for it came up. Instead, they decided to intervene, still as outside authorities, in situations where they really had no expertise. They had not addressed the original problem of mistrust and pessimism.

In order to design a new study, the nurses began by asking, "If these were not the people's most important problems, what should we ask? Where should we look? How can we recognize what the real problems are?"

With their anthropological training, they realized that the answer to these questions grows out of the basic purpose they have, as researchers, in asking the question. What people say about their problems may or may not be what the nurses were looking for. If they wanted to intervene in people's lives in order to improve their health, the "data" would grow out of a long, respectful dialogue between them and the villagers about what is wanted, how these wants are related to the lives of the people as a whole, and how the nurses' knowledge as health professionals can be added to theirs, in search of better health.

Once they had spent some time in the village observing everyday life, the nurse anthropologists began to realize two things: First, that fighting over loans meant that the system of interpersonal relationships as a whole in the village was under strain from new economic conditions; and second, that the villagers were very upset by conflict of any kind, and therefore they paid more attention to problems that generate conflict than to problems that do not. The nurse anthropologists considered that this sounds like an issue that might have long-term health effects, but wondered if it was the most critical one in the village. They also wondered what long-term impact the proposed solution would have on the whole complex of relationships in the village.

The nurse anthropologists also considered that the behavior of the youths was probably a symptom of the same combination of big changes in local culture plus a strong dislike of conflict. Only when the villagers themselves began to grasp and confront these deeper causes would they be able to make any lasting headway toward solving them, or even to decide whether or not this was really an important problem. Helping them do that would require a major change in the way the health professionals behaved toward them – a shift from remote and often critical authorities who had no knowledge of local affairs, to trusted participants in village life.

As the nurse anthropologists began to discuss these ideas with the villagers in order to clarify them, the villagers began to think more clearly about their own problems. Many of them began to realize that these problems were not as serious as the fact that social life in the village was being ruined by the new economic situation, which had divided families, alienated youth from their parents, and undermined cooperation between neighbors. They decided to form some new organizations that would discuss solutions to these problems.

Some of the public health authorities in the region had not been trained in anthropology, and they did not understand the value of the nurse anthropologists' view. They felt it simply was not "scientific." They wanted to know the "correct answer" to the question, "What do the villagers want?" But the nurse anthropologists said to them, "There is no correct answer to this question. Most of the villagers had probably not thought about the question carefully, and they might have changed their answers if they had some time to discuss it among themselves and think it over. The true answers will emerge out of this kind of interaction, in which the nurses simply help the villagers to think."

The idea that *science* consists of constructing a model or hypothesis, and then finding the correct data to test it, is the laboratory science way of thinking, and it is not applicable in this situation. During their first study, the nurse researchers' problem was that they had not learned to think of social knowledge in a new way, different from the laboratory-science method they had been taught throughout their careers. Once they had been trained to think as anthropologists, they began to look at social facts not as data based on a hypothesis — objective facts that one extracts from a situation and then analyzes, but as the *emerging product of a purposeful interaction between themselves and their clients.* This way of thinking, which I call the naturalistic theory, is a different, and equally sound, scientific theory of knowledge that I will explain in the next chapter.

THE LIMITS OF POSITIVISM

Because positivism is so useful, it is also very convincing, and even now is widely believed to be the best, or even the only valid, theory of how we know things scientifically. In the past hundred years, however, social scientists and philosophers have gradually discovered that positivism has very strict limitations as a practical theory of knowledge. A hundred years ago, many people believed that the new positivist sciences of psychology and sociology would allow humankind to develop models of how our minds and societies work – models so useful that we would soon be using them to design far better education systems, mental health practices, and even whole societies. But progress has been much slower than scientists hoped, and many new social problems have appeared that the positivists did not predict and so far have been unable to solve.

Why is this so? Apparently, things like minds and social systems are so complex and unstable that it is impossible, practically speaking, to design experiments that will allow us to develop generally useful positivist theories about them.[1] We cannot put a human community in a laboratory and expect it to function normally. Ethically, we cannot test social hypotheses by making people live their lives this way or that just so we can observe them. We have to use observations of life in natural communities, which means there are many, many things that we are not permitted to observe at all. It also means that we can rarely get agreement, even between trained observers, about what is actually happening in a social setting. So many things are going on at once that our perception necessarily depends on what we choose to ignore. Moreover, unlike the behavior of atoms or microbes, human behavior almost always provokes moral reactions in human observers, and there is no place for such reactions in positivist science.

When one tries to follow a positivist conception of science under these circumstances, several unfortunate things are likely to happen:

1. The selection of measurements that are suitably exact and stable, but whose relationship to the real purpose of the research is far from clear. For example, if we want to measure the effects of poverty on health, we can look at the income people report on their tax returns and other government documents as a measure of poverty. Asking people how much money they make might be subject to too much error. But without information on what other sources of livelihood people may have (such as informal cash income, gifts and favors, self-produced goods, etc.) and how they use their resources, one is not able to imagine accurately the relationship between the measure of income and the problem. Since it is impossible to collect reliable data on things that are

---

[1] There are those who argue that this problem does not disprove the truth of the positivist theory of knowledge. They argue that if we had the necessary recording and data processing capabilities, we could devise general and useful theories about these very complex things. This is an interesting argument but it is not relevant to my task, which is to offer a theory of knowledge that is useful *here and now* for understanding social systems.

really important in solving a particular research problem within the time frame and design of the study, researchers often construct hypotheses that they imagine can be tested with data that are easy to collect, and try to make sense out of this without getting anywhere near a useful answer to their problem. The *Ban Chan Village* example, given above, might be said to illustrate this.

2. The selection of measures that are relevant to the problem but are highly inexact and variable, which are then treated as though they were exact and stable. Continuing with the above example, self-reports about needs, for example, might turn out to be useful, but we cannot know how they are related to any *objective* measure of poverty. The *Ban Chan Village* example could also be used here. When people are asked to identify the most important problem in their village, they are likely to come up with some kind of answer, even if they have never thought about the issue at all and really have no opinion. But their answers are then given a knowledge status equal to something fairly measurable, such as of the number of married couples in the village or the rate of death by motor accidents.

3. If you begin with a hypothesis, you begin by assuming, for the sake of study, that the measures you will take are related to each other in a specific way, usually with some measures assumed to be *causing* others. Having discovered a statistical association between two measures, one is likely to assume that the hypothetical causal relationship between them is thereby confirmed. Without knowing the complexity of the situation, this inference might be completely false. An actual example of this is the discovery in the 1950s that there was a statistical correlation between poverty and rates of schizophrenic diagnosis. One is tempted to suppose that poverty contributes to susceptibility to the disease schizophrenia, or vice-versa, that having schizophrenia puts one at risk for poverty. But there are several completely different explanations that make just as much sense. For example, when the study in question was done, there was no reliable treatment for schizophrenia, and low-income victims were consigned to public institutions with a minimum of care. Therefore, if a penniless person saw a private psychiatrist, that psychiatrist would be motivated (perhaps unconsciously) to diagnose him or her schizophrenic, thereby solving the problem of who would pay for the treatment. A person with ample resources would be more likely to get (again, perhaps unconsciously) a different evaluation – a disease the therapist could treat and collect a fee for. In addition, people who live in low-income neighborhoods have far less privacy than those in middle

class neighborhoods, because housing is more crowded and there are more people in the streets. Also, the police visit low-income neighborhoods far more often than other ones. So, if a person is acting strangely in a poor district, they are more likely to be picked up by the police and diagnosed as mentally ill than those showing the same behavior in a middle class district.

As a result of these and other problems, most of the practical difficulties that have been addressed by the social sciences still remain to be solved. Many social scientists who work in a positivist way admit this, and they usually explain that social science is only about a century old, and their techniques just have to be refined. Obviously, I do not believe this is true. I believe that the laboratory-based model of knowledge is fundamentally the wrong model for understanding social life. I believe anthropologists must understand and use a different theory of knowledge – one that will allow them to achieve practical results, while still being able to claim that their results are valid in a scientific sense. In Chapter Three, we explore the *naturalistic theory of knowledge*, the anthropological way of knowing.

SUMMARY

The laboratory theory of knowledge is based on the idea that we can discover universal and permanent laws governing the way all things behave if we follow a certain exact procedure. This procedure requires us to break complex processes down into simple ones that can be measured accurately. This theory of knowledge is very useful for studying relatively simple processes, but it creates severe problems when we try to study very complex ones. We cannot isolate or measure exactly all the important processes that contribute to community health, for example. We must use another theory of truth that leads to practical results without requiring exactness. I call this theory the *naturalistic theory of knowledge*. At the same time, laboratory methods are extremely useful for some things, such as measuring the rates of disease in a community. For this reason, nearly all social science research actually uses a combination of laboratory-like and naturalistic methods.

CHAPTER THREE

The Naturalistic Theory of Knowledge: Anthropology

GUIDE TO THIS CHAPTER

In this chapter, I present the naturalistic theory of knowledge, which I believe to be more useful than positivism as a basic knowledge theory for the
social sciences. First, I outline the main features of the naturalistic theory
and discuss some reasons for preferring it to positivism as a social science
philosophy. Next, I discuss some common scientific ideas, such as theory-
building and verification, as they apply to the naturalistic theory. I refer to
research based on the naturalistic theory simply as *naturalistic research*.

NATURALISTIC THEORY

In the last hundred years or so, several prominent social scientists have
been concerned about the problems of trying to apply positivistic logic to
social systems, and have developed theories of knowledge that seek to deal
with those problems. I have learned much from the writings of Max Weber
(1962), John Dewey (1984), Júrgen Habermas (1978), C. Wright Mills
(1959), Barney Glazer and Anselm Strauss (1967), and Martyn Hammersley and Paul Atkinson (1995).[1] The theories of knowledge that they
developed for social science are often collectively called *pragmatism* – the
name that Dewey adopted for his method – but I prefer to call them *naturalistic theory*, because they closely resemble the way we human beings
ordinarily understand things and invent solutions in our everyday lives.

As a theory of knowledge, naturalistic theory proposes that:

1. There may or may not be an objective universe independent of our
   observation, but if so, we cannot know it as it is – we can only

---

[1] Hammersley and Atkinson (1995) trace the origin of the term *naturalism* to Lofland in
1967, and note that the term has also been used by Blumer, Denzin, and others.

know things as our senses (and sense-enhancing tools) present
them to us.

2. We can have practical knowledge of things, knowledge that helps
us accomplish our goals, without knowing the universe as it is.

3. All objective knowledge is in fact practical – it is the answer to
a question that a purposeful observer asks about something. In
other words, it is the solution to a problem.

4. Knowledge can be verified by applying it to real situations and
observing whether it solves the problems it was meant to solve,
where no contrary knowledge seems to explain the result better
than the knowledge we used.[2]

5. Human knowledge is never universal or timeless. It is temporary
and contingent, grounded in impermanent, possibly unique, real
situations.

The Idea of Usefulness

Key to the naturalistic theory of knowledge is the idea of *usefulness*,
or practicality, which needs some explaining. William James, the great
philosopher and psychologist who really invented pragmatism, understood this, and I rely heavily on his ideas (James, 1948). In ordinary
conversation, we usually say something is *useful* or practical if it helps
us accomplish some task. A useful tool makes work easier or the results
better. A useful idea helps us solve intellectual problems with practical
results. But James wanted the idea of usefulness to have a broader meaning. Claiming that all knowledge is practical requires us to recognize that
anything that helps to satisfy an urge to know of any kind can be called
useful or practical. The desire to make a chair or table produces an urge
to know the techniques and materials. The desire to raise good children
drives us to search for wise parenting methods. The desire to know why
one painting strikes us as more beautiful than another urges us to understand aesthetics. The wish to help others, or to deal justly with them,
leads us to seek understanding of their needs and desires, as well as to
develop principles of justice.

I believe a definition of knowledge based on this idea of usefulness
is completely in keeping with the so-called physical sciences. Many great
physicists have written about the process of discovery, and most agree

---

[2] Here I differ from Hammersley (2001), who proposes that naturalistic social science should
strive to describe a world somewhat independent of our judgment. Hammersley proposes
what he calls *subtle realism*, a knowledge in which we have "reasonable confidence," without
either pretending to have absolute truth, or accepting the hopeless relativism of the individual
understanding.

that it is a matter of searching for what James called *mental repose*, the feeling of pleasure that accompanies the certainty that we have satisfied our curiosity.

Throughout this book, I emphasize that good research always begins with an accurate statement of our urge to know. If the need is not clear, the search will be awkward and the results likewise unclear.

THE NATURALISTIC SEARCH FOR KNOWLEDGE

There are many methods for pursuing naturalistic knowledge. There is no single way to proceed. Some of the methods naturalistic researchers use resemble those that are used in positivist studies, but with a different meaning. What follows is my own attempt to make the process of naturalistic inquiry systematic and clear, and I agree that there are other possible ways of doing this.

Intuition, or Using What We Already Know

Unlike most writers on scientific method, I believe it is helpful to explain clearly how any such method relies on the large store of knowledge that any scientist already has before beginning a careful study of any subject. I am referring to the type of background knowledge we all rely on whenever we begin to solve a problem in everyday life. – I call this type of knowledge *intuition*.

Intuition is the loose arrangement of experience, observations, and thoughts that have some bearing on the problem we are setting out to study. These ideas and thoughts are usually vague and unclear at first. By focusing our attention on them, we are able to understand what more we need to know in order to have a clear idea of the thing we want to learn.

Here is an example of how each one of us uses intuition every day in our lives when we need to make a decision or carry out a plan. Suppose I want to buy a birthday present for my cousin George. In making a decision what to buy, first it is important to know what my goals are. First, buying a birthday present is a general situation that I have experienced many times, and I know from experience that:

1. I want George to enjoy what I give him.
2. I want to be able to give it to him on his actual birthday, not earlier or later.
3. I do not want to spend more money than I can reasonably afford, but I do not want to seem stingy by sending something too cheap.

With these goals, I begin to explore in my mind what I already know about the specific context, namely, what kind of person my cousin is, where he lives, and what he might like.

First, if he is to enjoy my present, it should have certain general qualities: (a) it should be something he does not already have; (b) it should be the type of thing he likes – it should suit his tastes and the way he lives; and, (c) it should be something he is able to use right away, without buying anything extra to use it. Again, thinking about the specific context of cousin George, I have a little bit of knowledge, not much, about what he has and what he likes. By reviewing this knowledge I can make some progress deciding what to buy. I do know that he has a CD player, and likes classical music, but I do not know what classical CDs he already has. I do not know his taste in clothes very well, so I might not buy him something unusual to wear. I do know that the winter is very cold in Chicago where he lives, and I also know that most men like to have several warm things to wear, so that they do not have to wear the same thing all the time. I do not know his favorite colors, but I think most men like to wear neutral colors, like tan or gray. I do not know exactly what size he wears, but I know he is about the same size as me, and I wear a size Medium. I have an intuition that he would like either a classical music CD, or something warm to wear, but still I am not sure about the details.

Next, I also know about his specific context that his birthday is on November 9th. I know it takes mail packages three days to reach Chicago. This means I must buy his present before, say, November 4th, in order to be sure he gets it on time.

Going back to the level of general knowledge, I know the typical amount to spend on a present for a cousin is less than $50, but more than $10. I can think about presents in this price range. As for this specific context, I do not know much about the prices of things, but I think a good overcoat costs more then $50, and I know that there is a discount clothing store near my house that sells nice looking sweaters for about $30. I know music CDs cost about $15 or $20. Because I live in California, I think I can buy wine more cheaply than my cousin can in Chicago, but I also know I cannot send wine in the mail, and anyway I don't know whether he likes wine.

Based on all this knowledge, there are several things I can do. I can call George's wife, to ask her what classical CDs he has and what his favorite colors are; or I can just select something *safe*, based on my limited knowledge. I decide to call his wife. When I call her, she tells me that he already has many sweaters, but he recently developed a taste for opera music, and has no CDs of that genre.

Based on this refinement of my intuition, I think some more. I know most people who like opera at all like Bizet's *Carmen*. I also know where

I can buy a recording of *Carmen*, and I know it is inexpensive to mail a CD; so, I decide that's what I will do. I now have a refined intuition that Cousin George will like a recording of *Carmen*, and that it will not cost too much, and I can get it in plenty of time for his birthday.

This kind of thinking that we all do every day is a very, very simple version of how one does research using the naturalistic method. Usually, we do not pay attention to the problem solving process itself, only on the answers. By making the process clearer, I have shown the basic steps of naturalistic research – only a more systematic and conscious version of what we already know how to do. The question is, why must naturalistic research be more conscious and systematic than ordinary problem solving?

How Science Is Different from Everyday Problem Solving: The Issue of *Persuasion*

If research were just the same as ordinary problem solving, we would not need a book that explains how to do it. The big difference between the two is that one of the purposes of research is to change the way other people think about the problem – to persuade other people to think seriously about our solution. This is true not just of the naturalistic method, but of all scientific research. We can say that science itself is a set of rules about what is, and is not, persuasive to scientists. Of course, because science has very high prestige in modern societies, ideas gain general persuasive power in those societies if scientists accept them.

As I mentioned when I discussed scientific method in the first two chapters, persuasion in science depends on the researcher being able to explain in detail how the conclusions were reached. One has to show one's fellow scientists just what was done in order to arrive at the results, and convince them that if they did the same thing, they would reach the same conclusions. In other words, while we seldom have to explain how we solved a particular problem in everyday life (especially if the solution is a good one!), in science, we must *make the entire problem solving process itself conscious, and document it.*

THE PROCESS OF NATURALISTIC RESEARCH

We are now ready to state simply the overall process of research using the naturalistic method, as follows:

1. We begin not with a theory or model, but with a practical problem – a situation that must be understood in order to reach

a specific goal. It is important to be able to state the problem precisely, because every step of the inquiry must be guided by a sense of what kind of solution is needed. In order to state the problem precisely, one must have clear knowledge of one's own subjective values about the inquiry. (That is, why does one want to solve this problem?)

2. We devise a careful *guess*, or an intuition about what the answer to the problem might look like *in* the context of the situation we want to understand.

3. We bring together and clarify as much as possible all the knowledge we already have about the problem, the context, and the intuition.

4. We then search this knowledge to find the gaps: what observations are necessary in order to test the intuition – to fill in the missing pieces of the solution, and find out whether the pieces we have intuited are accurate (that is, useful) or not?

5. We devise whatever methods are called for to get the missing information. In order to be scientific, these methods must be persuasive – other scholars and relevant laymen must be able to imagine using them, and feel that they are sensible. Our most important method is *participant observation*, taking part in the everyday social setting we want to understand, in order to learn how it works as a whole.

6. Each piece of information we get this way is continuously compared with the original intuition, to see if it fits. The intuition is modified or strengthened accordingly. We might even throw the intuition out and start over.

7. The modified intuition then suggests new questions to ask, and steps (5)and (6) are repeated, until either we run out of time, or until we are more or less satisfied with the answer, and satisfied that we can show how we reached it.

I will come back to these steps and discuss them thoroughly in the chapters on methods. Now I want to say something about the advantages of the naturalistic theory of knowledge and the method it generates.

ADVANTAGES OF NATURALISTIC KNOWLEDGE

Several features of naturalistic knowledge make it especially useful, particularly in the health sciences. These advantages are most clearly seen in the issues of *meaning* and *pattern coherence*.

The Issue of Meaning

Science recently has made great strides toward predicting complex processes like the weather, using brilliant inventions like satellite videography and high-speed computer analysis. But we are still a long way from being able to predict the weather perfectly, even though it adheres to thoroughly tested physical laws. And we are much, much farther from being able to predict the behavior of human groups or individuals. One reason for this is that human behavior is not guided by physical events per se, but by the *meanings* people attach to events, and the process of attaching meanings does not follow a mechanical cause-and-effect pattern. Rather: (a) it is *experience based*, which means it varies from person to person, group to group, and day to day; (b) it is *contextual*, that is, the meaning one attaches to any thing or event is highly dependent on the whole configuration of things, events and the meanings that surround it; and worst of all, (c) meaning formation is *creative*, in the sense that people can and do make up new meanings for things as they go along – meanings that have never been attached to those things before.

EXAMPLE: Mrs. Ito and the Nurse

Years ago I was studying the status of the elderly in Japanese American culture. Among other things, I wanted to know how the experience of growing old was different in Euro-American and Japanese American cultures, including the sources of difficulty and the sources of satisfaction. This question in turn was meant to give me a richer understanding of the role played by cultural patterns such as kinship, religion, and values, in determining the well-being of elderly people in my own culture.

I learned that almost all Japanese immigrants at that time had come to America prior to 1924. They had come from a Japan that had been nearly isolated from the world for three centuries, and they were quite unsophisticated about other races and cultures. Never having seen a person of African ancestry until they arrived here, most were simply afraid of African Americans whom they did not know personally. The two groups were extremely different both physically and culturally. The immigrants were used to a highly formal, quiet, deferential social atmosphere, and did not know what to make of the African American style, which tends to be just the opposite – spontaneous, emotional, emphatic. To make matters worse, many Japanese immigrants had trouble with English, and often could not understand the accents of people from the American Deep South – this was especially true of the Japanese women, who had little formal education even in their own language.

During my research I learned that a woman I knew, an immigrant in her 80s I'll call Mrs. Ito, had broken her hip and was in the hospital. I knew that hospitalization is a common experience of old people, and I thought this would be a good opportunity to start filling a hole in my intuition about sources of stress and satisfaction: What different difficulties and possibilities does hospitalization produce in the two cultures?

When I went to visit Mrs. Ito in her hospital room, I found her sitting up in bed, alone and inattentive to her surroundings. She had the television on but was not watching it, having lost her glasses. Mrs. Ito did not speak English anyway, but at least she could have had something to look at. A tray of typical hospital food (very un-Japanese) sat untouched beside her.

I was feeling uncomfortable, thinking she must be quite lonely and bored, when into the room came one of her nurses, a very large African American woman. "Momma!" the nurse bellowed, bustling around her bed, "What are we going to do with you? You haven't touched your lunch!" Her tone was half-joking, half-scolding – a tone that I doubted Mrs. Ito could interpret. I winced. What could it have been like for her to be here in this totally unfamiliar setting, separated from family, friends, language, and culture, and attended by someone she was afraid of?

At that moment, Mrs. Ito turned to me and smiled. In Japanese she said, "She calls me 'Momma,' like my children do." Then she lay back peacefully, and I could see that she was in fact quite comfortable, perhaps even happy.

On my way home I remembered that in Japanese culture, illness is often understood not as a time of suffering, or even of boredom. Rather it is one of the few times when people are free of their heavy social obligations, and can expect to be entirely passive and pampered, almost always by female kin. There were two nearly opposite sets of meanings Mrs. Ito could have readily attached to the African American nurse – the frightening, big, loud stranger, or the warm, nurturing daughter-substitute. She had chosen the latter. For her part, the nurse may have known little about Japanese culture, but she knew the universal meaning of the word, "Momma."

As for me, I reflected that I was raised in a culture where race is always a major factor in any interaction between strangers of different colors, and I had overreacted, projecting my own sensitivity onto the situation. I wondered if Mrs. Ito could just have easily chosen the racial meaning. If I had been asked before this incident about the wisdom of assigning African American nurses to elderly Japanese immigrant patients, I would have recommended against it, but afterward I would have said, "I don't know whether race is an important factor."

What if I had tried to answer the question about the impact of racial attitudes on the health of the elderly immigrants by quasi-laboratory methods? What if I had constructed opinion questionnaires based on the hypothesis that Japanese patients would not want to be treated by African American personnel? I would have had to be very lucky, or very clever, to understand that other features of the social context may be more important than race, and something about why, and this might have had major practical implications for the research. I would have been likely to measure the wrong thing, and it would have been very difficult to discover the mistake.

To understand a system that is built up out of subjective meanings like this, the idea of hypotheses based on universal laws is an awkward idea. One cannot predict at all accurately what meanings key people will attach to key events. One needs a locally valid model of meaning-formation, otherwise one is at a loss either to predict what will happen with any accuracy, or to interpret what did happen.

Through the research process I have described, one can often arrive at useful knowledge that fits the situation at hand. By participating in the interpretive process, one observes regularities and variations in the ways individuals and groups of people make meaning, and the consequences of that process. In the example of *Mrs. Ito and the Nurse*, my naturalistic research on the Japanese American aged was greatly enriched by this single incident. Later I was able to observe other settings where the meaning of race was superceded by other meanings, and settings where it was not. I began to develop a sense of the flexibility of this meaning.

If I had started out the study by forming hypotheses about the two cultures and trying to test these hypotheses with exact measurements that could have been repeated by other researchers, the outcome would have been very different. I probably would not have thought about putting race relations into my measurements to begin with. If I had thought of it, I would have had serious trouble trying to devise measures of racial meanings that could be replicated in other studies. And even if I had found such measures, I would probably not have learned about the ways in which racial meanings are situational in Japanese American life, and how they can simply be overwhelmed by other meanings. I return to the issue of meaning and context in Chapter Four.

The Issue of Pattern Coherence

As soon as anthropologists began studying actual living societies by living in them and observing then systematically (in the late nineteenth century), they noticed the close interdependence of the various parts of the local culture. Economic activity, art and folklore, technology, science and magic, kinship, politics and law, religion, and sexuality were all intimately related. They seemed to fit together into a pattern, and a change in one part of the pattern could easily disrupt other parts, even setting off a cascade of changes that threatened the integrity of the whole system. In Chapter One I gave the example of how economic and technological changes in rural Thailand set off such a catastrophic process.

This means it is nearly impossible to target a small area of behavior – such as health practices, for example – and predict how that part will change under specified conditions, such as the introduction of new knowledge or technology. Rather, what is needed to solve human problems is a very wide knowledge of the entire system of belief, activity, and environment of which the targeted behavior is an integral part. Operating with a positivist theory of knowledge, this would mean we could not approach any social problem scientifically – we could not validate our propositions – unless we could get experts to agree on at least a rough description of where our hypothesis fits in the whole system. This is completely impractical, because social systems are so complex that scholars rarely agree on how to describe them. With a naturalistic knowledge theory, it is not necessary for scholars to agree – they only have to be willing to see whether our description of the system is useful for the purposes at hand – whether it is persuasive and not directly contradictory to others' factual knowledge on the most critical points.

Turn again to the example of *Ban Chan Village*, given in Chapter Two. The nurses wanted to get a description of the villagers' beliefs that could not be challenged, that was not biased by the preconceptions of the researchers, or by faulty data collection methods. They had followed all the positivistic procedures of questionnaire construction – pre-testing, validity and reliability checks, and so on. Thanks to this preoccupation, at first they failed to focus on the way their data was dependent on its social and historical context. In order to focus on the larger pattern that was needed to interpret their data, the nurses finally had to spend a lot of time observing life in the village. They had to think creatively about models that might predict the effects of any intervention. Before they studied anthropology, this kind of work seemed unacceptably subjective to them, because each observer would see different things and describe them differently.

If the naturalistic theory of knowledge can accept alternative descriptions of a single social system, is it then hopelessly subjective? Does it mean that anyone can devise a description of their own and claim it is *true* because it produces results? The answer is, anyone can try, but their description will not be widely accepted unless it persuades others, often including the people they are studying, who have experience with the system as well. Consider two things:

First, because human social systems are so complex, if you are going to convince anyone who has considerable experience of a system that you have understood it, you had better know a great deal about it first. Second, if you study the way positivistic science is actually performed, you will find that persuasion plays a very large role there, too.

If several studies produce different results, which study is the most reliable? If several interpretations of a finding are not contradicted by the available data, which one do you choose? You must often persuade your colleagues that you have made the most sensible choice, and it is often a matter of how clearly you explain your method, and how well you document it, not a matter of the data themselves, in determining which choice is best.

THE DISADVANTAGES OF NATURALISTIC THEORY

For all its advantages, naturalistic theory does pose several conceptual and practical problems for the researcher. These problems are discussed in more detail in Chapter Thirteen, where we discuss the slightly different conceptions of professionalism in the health sciences and the naturalistic social sciences. Here, let us look at the most important kinds of objections positivist scientists raise when evaluating naturalistic research results.

Conceptual Problem No. 1: Verification

Naturalistic accounts are always the product of a unique relationship between one or more scholar-observers on one hand, and the people being observed on the other. The method requires: (a) detailed observation and recording of actual sequences of natural human events; and, (b) intensive participation by the researchers in the everyday life of the observed people. By its nature, the resulting data are unique to the specific study, and cannot be very closely reproduced by other scholars, or even by the same scholars in another time and place. In other words, the data of *naturalistic studies cannot be verified in some of the ways that experimental data can be* – for example, by repeating the experiment, or one very similar. As a result, using the positivist canons of the experimental sciences, there may not be a clear way to choose among two or more naturalistic accounts that disagree with one another. To make such a judgment, one must rely on indications of the researcher's depth of familiarity with the study material, and his or her powers of persuasion, as to the correctness of the interpretation. I call this the *problem of verification.*

For example, I can test the effectiveness of a particular medicine for a particular disease by using the experimental method of a randomized, double-blind trial. You probably know how this works. As experimental subjects, I recruit a group of people who have certain characteristics that are considered to have an effect on the disease in question. I carefully document these "patients'" characteristics (age, gender, health status, and so on). I assign equal numbers of these subjects to three groups: a *drug therapy* group, a *placebo* group, and a *no intervention* group. I do this in such a way that neither the researchers nor the subjects themselves know (at first) who is in which group. After the intervention, I measure the outcome – what happened to all of the subjects. If those who got the medicine had statistically better outcomes than those who got either the placebo or nothing, I think I have shown the effectiveness of the medicine. Any other trained experimenter can do this same procedure and check to see if the results are the same. If they are, I can say the study has been validated. If they are not, I can check the methods of the two studies, to make a new hypothesis about why the results were different, and do another experiment to test this new hypothesis.

Now let us take a naturalistic science example. Suppose I want to see whether a particular kind of incentive (let's say, giving people a good citizen award) will get subjects to reduce their blood pressure with diet, exercise, and abstinence from smoking. I can do a randomized trial, but it cannot be double blind, because obviously the patients will know what they did. Moreover, if the incentive group gets better results than the no incentive group, I do not know *why*. Was it because they wanted the incentive, or because they wanted to please this particular researcher, or because people in this particular community worry about the social consequences of failure, or something else? If someone else tries to repeat my experiment and gets different results, does that mean there were social or psychological differences between the two samples, or that something about public attitudes had changed between the two studies, or that the different personalities of the researchers affected the subjects in different ways? There must be some other standard than agreement that will allow us to judge the results of the study.

Conceptual Problem No. 2: Objectivity

The second conceptual problem has to do with the fact that human systems are the product of thought, and thought cannot be directly observed, it must be inferred from its results. Naturalistic social science evolved as a method in the first place in response to the discovery that human behavior in groups is not the result of a series of mechanical reactions to measurable facts. Rather, thought and judgment make the *reality* that different people are viewing look different to them. Action, as we say, is always mediated by an interpretive process – a culturally patterned, often unconscious way of assigning meaning and value to things, whose function can only be understood by observing its consequences. People do not act directly on an objectively real environment; they act on a perceived environment, the perception of which is largely shaped by their culture. They *socially construct* their world (Berger & Luckman, 1967). This extremely valuable point of view puts the observer in a curious place with respect to the idea of universal truth: Since social research itself is an expression of cultural behavior, it cannot be said to represent objective reality any more than the human beliefs which it describes. Philosophically, one must either reject social construction as a principle, or accept the fact that one's own naturalistic studies are not evidence of some universal reality, but are social constructions also (Hammersley, 1995). If one chooses the latter, of course the problem arises of explaining how one's own naturalistic science account can be more scientific than other kinds of accounts – accounts based on folklore, for example (Cochran, 2002). I call this the *problem of objectivity*.

Scientific findings are of little use unless their validity is widely accepted by those who might use them. A health professional who wants to use naturalistic methods needs to have a clear grasp of these two problems – *verification* and *objectivity* – and their solutions, in order convince other health professionals that such methods produce useful results.

The Naturalistic Response

In the naturalistic theory of knowledge, the test of the validity and reliability of one's data is whether it can be used to solve problems, not whether the same relationships among measures can be generated at different times, or by different researchers, or in different populations using the same techniques. In the positivist approach, the basic idea is that there is one *correct* set of data, and all other sets are *incorrect*. One's method should be able to eliminate, or at least minimize, the latter. In the naturalistic approach, there can be various "correct" ways of looking at things, as there are various ways to solve a given problem. It is helpful to be able to explain incompatible findings, but the incompatibility itself does not invalidate them.

In practice, there is often not so much difference between the positivistic and the naturalistic kinds of validity and reliability. If I ask ambiguous questions so that I cannot use the answers to solve a problem, the naturalist can say my data are not valid or reliable. The positivist can say the same thing, if my ambiguous data do not show the predicted consistent, coherent pattern.

There is also a good deal of overlap in the way validity and reliability can be tested *in process* in the two approaches to knowledge. Both may have different observers look at the same phenomena, or ask the same questions. Both may use *triangulation*, asking the same basic questions in a variety of different ways, and from a variety of different kinds of respondents.

In the matter of validity and reliability, anthropological method has two very great advantages over quasi laboratory method. First, the researcher immerses herself in the community under study, and constantly checks previous observations against new ones. Accordingly, she is likely to detect unhelpful conclusions early on, and be able to modify them. Second, the researcher observes things in their natural context and constantly reflects on the relationships between them. Accordingly, she is likely to be able to figure out *why* her observations were unhelpful, and correct her method accordingly.

EXAMPLE: Tepoztlán, Two Villages in One

In the 1920s, anthropologist Robert Redfield wanted to find out whether there are basic similarities among peasant villages in different parts of the world. He went to the state of Morelos, in Mexico, where he lived in and studied a village he called Tepoztlán. There, Redfield found a great many forms of cooperation among the village families, forms that are weak or missing in large urban settings. There were cooperative work groups, festivals and rites, political alliances, and religious ties of many kinds. Based on this, and on his own and other anthropologists' work, Redfield (1930) concluded that peasant society in general is rich in these cooperative structures.

In the 1940s, another famous anthropologist, Oscar Lewis (1951), was also interested in the matter of conflict and cooperation among economically marginal people in all kinds of societies, urban as well as rural. He decided to go to Tepoztlán and take another look. In contrast to what Redfield saw, Lewis found a lot of evidence of strife and conflict in the village – fights and feuds, insults, lawsuits, even murder. He wondered if the village had changed in the past 20 years, but court records and people's memories said it had not.

Must we conclude that either Redfield or Lewis, or both, did a poor job of finding the facts in Tepoztlán? I would say no. Each of them began with a specific problem: Redfield was interested in how people in technologically simple societies manage to get along together and make a living. Lewis was interested in what poverty does to people, regardless of other features of their way of life. Each of them discovered part of the truth about Tepoztlán, and each of them made important contributions to our knowledge, not only about Tepoztlán, but also about human behavior in general. Since their work, other anthropologists have been able to use Redfield and Lewis's work to understand a host of similar problems. (See Ingham, 1986)

In short, the naturalistic theory of knowledge, and this book, suggest that questions of validity and reliability should ask, not "are the data *correct?*" in some absolute sense, but "are the data *persuasive* and *useful* in this context, for this problem?" Now we are ready to begin looking at the naturalistic research process itself.

Practical Problem No. 1: Time

The *practical* obstacles to the wider acceptance of naturalistic social science may be even greater. First, it is based on the notion that social systems are integrated wholes, that no particular behavior can be correctly understood in isolation from the full pattern, or system, of which it is a part. The meaning of acts can be shown to change according to their setting, actors, and antecedents. In practice, what this means is that, no matter how limited or specific the research problem, the researcher must sample a wide range of behaviors, often extending over months and involving dozens or even hundreds of incidents and actors, in order to begin to grasp clearly the larger patterns of which the research problem is a part. Briefly, there is no quick and simple way to do adequate naturalistic studies (*cf.* May & Pope, 2000, p. 52; Ten Have, 2004, p. 12). This often creates a problem for health researchers trying to work within the schedules of bureaucratic health organizations. Accountability in such organizations generally requires frequent reports that give, if not the solutions of concrete problems, at least a road map showing how progress toward these solutions is being made. The amassing of raw field notes over a period of years may not satisfy such requirements. I call this the *problem of time.*

Look again at the blood pressure control example: if I really want to know why my incentive worked or did not work, as an anthropologist I can spend a lot of time in the neighborhood where I am doing the study. I can observe what people do, ask them what they think and feel about it, talk to their families and neighbors, and try to understand how they live and how they make sense out of the whole hypertension issue. This way, I can devise a subtle explanation that takes into account many things that might have an effect, such as what it means to these people to be healthy, what kinds of foods they like and why, what it means to get this or that kind of award, what kinds of economic pressure they felt for or against the program, and so on. The more time I spend in the neighborhood, the better I get to know the people and their environment, the more confident I can be about understanding the results. At some point I will have to produce a report, but the quality of the report will increase with the depth of my experience, and a few weeks or months probably will not be enough to do a good job.

Practical Problem No. 2: Generalizability

As a second practical difficulty (related to the first, and to the conceptual problem of verification), is that the knowledge naturalistic social science produces cannot be applied widely outside the settings where it was produced, without careful restudy and modification. The very usefulness of naturalistic research is that it traces out the interconnections among the specific objects of interest (for example, hypertension rates in a population, or the impact of a needle exchange program) and the whole configuration of culture, economics, environment, politics, and history that together determine why people think and behave the way they do, and why they get the results they do. Since these complex configurations are unique to time and locale, the possibility of applying the findings of one study to other times and locales is always problematic. This of course does not mean that progress is impossible through naturalistic social science. It does, however, limit the practical expertise of the researcher to those times and locales that he or she actually knows fairly intimately. Although one might argue that this rule ought to be applied to all social knowledge, that does not solve the practical problem: In the existing social world of health science (and I believe this is true everywhere), the advancement of the researcher often depends on his or her ability to produce widely applicable, highly portable knowledge. I call this the *problem of generalizability*.

Look again at our blood pressure control example. Suppose I spend several months in the neighborhood, applying good anthropological methods. I might be able to write a pretty convincing report to explain what happened. *But*: I cannot be at all sure that someone who follows the same logic in another community will get similar results, because no two communities contain the same personalities, or have identical histories, or attach the same meanings to the same acts, or experience the same economic pressures. In fact, it is unlikely that something that works in one neighborhood will work in another one where the conditions are different; and if it does not work, we must conduct a new study to find out why.

WHAT ABOUT THEORY?

What is the relationship between the naturalistic theory of knowledge, and the construction and use of theories of human society? I have said that the naturalistic knowledge model does not answer the question of whether there are eternal laws operating in the universe, independent of our observations. I have also said that truth, or validity, is considered by the naturalistic theory to be dependent on context, and temporary. Does this mean that we cannot build general theories that can be applied to new places and problems? To think so would seem to imply that the idea of *progress* in social science is an illusion – that we must start over anew each time we formulate a problem.

The naturalistic theory of knowledge allows us to both produce and use general theories of human behavior. Theories often provide much of the raw material for the intuitions that guide data collection (steps 2, 6, and 7 of the research process outlined on p. 40). If, for example, we are interested in helping a community to develop its own capacity for health promotion, we would be interested in theories that explain cooperation and conflict in communities, theories of individual motivation that explain why people do volunteer work, theories of how people learn new behaviors, and so on. These theories would be described as part of our original intuition about where to look for the answer to our problem, and they would be subject to refinement by our research. Note, however, that: (1) it is rare for a single theory to inform the starting intuition; and (2) the intuition usually includes ideas and models that are not part of the existing relevant theoretical literature on the problem, that are assembled on-the-spot, out of the researcher's experience of the particular situation of the research.

As a result of naturalistic research, the theories that formed part of the original intuition may be refined, discarded, or provisionally confirmed. I say *provisionally* confirmed in order to point out that confirmation by a single study, or even by several studies, does not lead the naturalistic researcher to conclude that the theories in question are universally valid. An example of an existing theory I have used in my own naturalistic research is Durkheim's theory of anomie, which I discuss again in detail in Chapter Ten. The use of this theory emerged as a way of explaining my own observations on community organizing.

Naturalistic research can also generate new general statements about social behavior, usually of the sort that sociologists call *middle range* theories (Glazer & Strauss, 1967). An example, in fact, is given in this book – the theoretical model I call *people meeting needs in patterned context*. This model grew out of several research projects I did over many years, using a naturalistic theory of knowledge. I simply put it together from approaches that seemed useful in a wide variety of settings, and then began to use it as part of my starting intuition in working on new problems. One uses such models to develop a list of questions and observations one needs in order to begin doing research. In a sense, you can say you are *testing* the model, or theory, but that is not the point of the research. Rather, the model will be altered, refined, or discarded according to whether it helps solve the problem or not.

SUMMARY

Anthropological research follows the *naturalistic theory of knowledge*, which contrasts with positivism by proposing that *knowledge* is always a useful answer to a question. *Useful* means that it satisfies a personal desire to know. Naturalistic knowledge is not absolute or independent of the observer; it is always dependent on the observer's needs, and on the local and temporary situation being observed.

Anthropological research is particularly useful for getting answers to questions about human social systems. Such systems are extremely complex, they change constantly, and they differ from place to place; so that our understanding must be grounded in a situation. Also, human systems do not operate according to mechanical laws, but grow organically out of the understandings and behaviors of the people who create and use them. Anthropological methods show us how to observe this creative process as it actually works, giving us useful understandings of how situations are related to outcomes.

The process of naturalistic research is a simple refinement of the way we ordinarily solve problems in everyday life. It begins with a common sense intuition of the answer to a practical question. This intuition allows us to think of what kinds of things to observe, and what kinds of questions to ask. By observing and asking *systematically*, we are able to *persuade* others that we have understood the problem in a useful way; and it is this ability to persuade that distinguishes anthropological science from everyday problem solving.

CHAPTER FOUR

The Study of Real People in Natural Situations

GUIDE TO THIS CHAPTER

The main purpose of this chapter is to describe the set of basic attitudes and assumptions that form the intellectual framework for doing anthropological research. In doing anthropology, one tries to understand as much as possible about the entire scope of shared beliefs and behavior in a group, not simply from the perspective of the outsider or professional, but as the people themselves understand it. It is a type of research that: (a) brings the researcher into the intimate lives of strangers, requiring sensitivity and responsibility; (b) exposes to the study community the researcher's own lack of knowledge, requiring humility and patience; (c) reveals to the researcher things about her own thinking that might be surprising or even disturbing, requiring maturity and self-confidence.

Here we also discuss the way human beings attach different meanings to things depending on the situation, or context, in which they are found. An important part of the research attitude is to avoid making conclusions about local understanding, until one has a sense of how situations can change that understanding.

ETHNOGRAPHY AND THE ANTHROPOLOGICAL ATTITUDE

The attitude of the practical anthropologist toward his or her work is different from that of a positivist researcher. The latter has a tendency to view himself as a highly trained expert, who carries an elite knowledge about social systems, a knowledge not shared by the people he studies. He often views his research subjects mainly as sources of scientific data – data that the subjects themselves cannot understand or use. He usually views his results as something to be shared directly with his scientific colleagues, and only indirectly, if at all, with the research community itself.

The anthropologist, by contrast, thinks of himself as a student of the people he studies. He considers that the subjects of his research are themselves the real experts in their own culture, and carry the answers he needs in order to understand them. He believes that if the knowledge he gains is accurate and useful, his research community should be able to understand it and use it (within the limits of their ability for self-reflection and change).

In this chapter we reflect on the relationship between these very different attitudes toward the research community on one hand, and two other characteristics of anthropology: (1) the anthropological way of knowing human societies – as integrated wholes that make sense to the people we are studying; (2) the way anthropologists work – living with a community for a fairly long time, and playing as natural a role as possible in their lives. In short, if you strive to know a human community the way the people who live there know it, you must try to experience life the way they experience it. And in order to do this, you must develop a relationship with your study community that will allow you to look at it very closely indeed, without disrupting it too much. As a natural consequence of this way of working, the anthropologist develops a relationship with the people he studies that looks more like a partnership, or even a friendship, than the positivist relationship of *outside expert* and *study subjects*.

The Moral Relationship of Researcher and Community

In a well-known article, anthropologist Clifford Geertz tells a story about a cockfight in a Balinese village he was studying. At a moment of high excitement, the police raided the illegal event, and the spectators fled. Geertz found himself running down a back alley with several villagers and scrambling over a wall to get away (Geertz, 1972). Of course it was unlikely that the police would have arrested the American professor, but his spontaneous and highly undignified behavior ended up helping him in his research – it showed the villagers that he was not as different from them as he looked. The incident is a good illustration of how anthropologists work, and why their attitude toward research differs from that of other professions.

Every long-lasting human social group has its own unique shared habits of perceiving, thinking, valuing, and doing. For this reason, it is often extremely difficult for people from one social group to understand and cooperate with those of another. History offers an endless series of tragedies and comedies that result from this fact. The great beauty of anthropology is that it seeks to explain human behavior in everyday terms that make these different ways of thinking and living clear and understandable to one another. Anthropologists try to use the concepts of one culture, usually their own, to describe as accurately as possible the everyday concepts, feelings, and habits of another; that is, to present the entire way of life and thinking of an unfamiliar social group as a complex but more or less unified pattern that *makes sense* to the people who live it. Since human life is never that tidy, the anthropologist also identifies things about individual lives that do not fit the pattern, and therefore do not make sense in these lives, and he explains why.

In order to do this successfully, anthropologists find that they must live and work as closely as possible to the people they are studying, and they must do this for relatively long periods of time. A year or more is the standard duration of a complete community study, and many anthropologists return to the same community again and again over many years. Only by observing behavior in a wide variety of settings, talking to many different kinds of people, and studying a great variety of activities, can the researcher begin to see the pattern that makes the whole way of life sensible to those who live it. Also, one knows that if one interrupts people's normal everyday lives too much, one might actually change the way they understand and do things. Taking tests and answering strange questions might be something unfamiliar to people. It is often better to spend one's time trying to understand through participation, observation, and natural conversation. Another kind of distortion results when strangers intrude into private situations, or ask questions about private things not shared outside the group. One must try to become familiar to the people one works with, and fit easily into the things they do. The anthropologist must try to fit herself into the pattern of people's lives as best she can.

Within this method, the difficulty, even impossibility, of remaining a *neutral* observer, whose personal relationship with the study community has little or no effect on the results of the study, can be illustrated by an example from a particularly productive research relationship – a type of relationship, by the way, that is quite common in anthropology.

EXAMPLE: Mrs. Kondo: "Facts" Reflect Research Relationships

Years ago I spent a year and a half in Japan, trying to understand how life in the new style apartment cities called new towns was affecting Japanese thought and behavior. I lived close to one of these new towns, and spent most of every day there, and many evenings as well, talking with the residents and taking part in activities. There were few men there in the daytime, but I got to know some of the women very well.

One of these women became my favorite source of information, and I visited her several times a week. I will call her Mrs. Kondo. She and her husband were about forty years old, and they had two children. Life in their tiny apartment was extremely cramped. In the early stages of my research, I asked Mrs. Kondo why she and her husband had chosen to live here. They were somewhat older than the average resident, and seemed to have more money and status as well.

Mrs. Kondo told me that she and her husband were determined to provide everything possible for their two children – an excellent education, music lessons, travel, and so on. She said that they could afford to live in more luxurious surroundings, but then it would be harder to provide these things.

As the weeks passed and we spoke of many things, it was always hard to ignore the seeming misfit between this life style and her age, status, and background. Several months into my research, she revealed something shameful to me – that she was not on speaking terms with her mother-in-law. She and her husband had been living in his parents' home before moving to the new town, but she had found the woman so unpleasant that she had simply left, as she said, "without even putting my shoes on," and telephoned her husband, saying she would not go back to the house. Any other place, she said, indicating the tiny apartment around her, was preferable.

A few more weeks of regular conversation passed, and Mrs. Kondo and I became quite comfortable in each other's company. Our relationship had become rather deep and complex. Now she was not just my key informant, we were, in a sense, friends. She felt free to discuss her anxieties and disappointments, to complain about her neighbors and tell their secrets, and even to reveal a sin or two of her own. One day she told me, quite naturally in the course of our conversation, that all was not well between her and her husband. She had told me earlier that he worked long hours and spent a lot of time with his male friends playing mah jongg, rarely coming home before late at night. Now, she revealed that she felt humiliated living here in this new town, with people who were of lower status than she was. The choice of housing was a calculated punishment her husband was inflicting on her for failing to get along with his mother.

These conversations with Mrs. Kondo greatly deepened my understanding of new town life. I began to understand how sensitive people were to social class markers, in a place where people had identical homes. I began to see that this was not just a new form of housing, but also a new form of social suffering that could be used in the exercise of power; and I gained knowledge of the power dynamics of Japanese middle-class marriage and family.

These insights were made possible by the complexity of our relationship. Mrs. Kondo had taken on a role as my helper and teacher (also helping me with my language), and I had reciprocated by listening sympathetically, by providing her some comic relief with my bad Japanese and awkward manners, and by small favors such as rides in my car. Our relationship had evolved gradually into a kind of intimacy that rewarded her with emotional release, and me with privileged views of her life.

The enterprise of trying to describe how people understand their own lives necessarily gives the anthropologist a very special relationship to her work and to the people she studies, in several ways. For one thing, she must be trusted in the settings where she works, and that trust must be earned – by showing respect, adhering to local rules, keeping her knowledge confidential, not taking sides or picking favorites, keeping her word, and doing what is expected of her. For another, the anthropologist often works in situations where everyone else present has far more relevant knowledge and ability than she does. In these situations, her understanding will be confused, her actions clumsy and inappropriate, her questions childish. Here the anthropologist puts herself in the role of the beginning student, and places the people around her – even if they are children or outcasts – in the role of patient, wise teachers.

The attitude needed to put an anthropologist in such situations is one of profound curiosity, a frame of mind where the urge to answer questions is stronger than the urge to avoid embarrassment, influence others, or win favors. Curiosity is a state of mind in which values and assumptions are put aside – temporarily at least – so the anthropologist can find value and meaning in the discovery of her surroundings as they present themselves.

Clearly these are rational strategies for doing good work, but they are not *merely* strategies. They require a certain profound view of the self and the human world on the part of the researcher if they are to be successful. As one begins to understand the logic and the pattern that underlies a way of life, one cannot fail to be genuinely impressed by its intricacy, its ancient origins, its effectiveness in meeting people's needs, even the creativity and individuality it allows the individual participant. Some elements of the culture under study might always remain morally or artistically unacceptable to the researcher. Moreover, the anthropologist thinks of every cultural pattern as, in some important ways, unique. One might have spent many years studying this village or tribe or city, but upon entry into a new setting, there will always be many important things one does not know. There is always much more to know than one can discover in a lifetime. The more one understands, the more one finds that is both admirable and puzzling.

In addition, unless the researcher is a consummate actor, it is too difficult to live pleasantly among a people for long without liking and respecting at least some of them. In order to do this, one must find some good in people's way of thinking and behaving.

The seasoned anthropologist, then, usually sees herself not as a holder of superior knowledge, but as an eternal student of life; approaching her people not with judgment, but with curiosity, and usually with a great deal of personal affection resulting from shared experience. An intimate familiarity with people's views of themselves and the world naturally leads to empathy as well as intellectual understanding. Like any good scientist, the anthropologist feels an obligation to the truth in a scholarly sense, but unlike many other scientists, the anthropologist also feels a strong moral obligation to the subjects under study – again, not just in an abstract sense, but in the same sense that any sane person feels obligated to friends and acquaintances. Holding intimate knowledge about people, and being trusted by them, places upon all of us the burden of conscience. We may not need to care *for* them, but we must care *about* them. Our judgments and actions toward them must be informed by our sense of justice and dignity, not just our assessment of facts.

Given this perspective, anthropologists are generally more comfortable with research projects in which the role of the researcher is defined as that of an advisor, participant, and collaborator, rather than as a neutral observer, or as the alien agent of a remote scientific community. In this sense, the researcher is inclined to want the research subjects to set the research agenda, ask the questions, and decide how to apply the results, while he observes, records, and feeds back information.

SURVEY RESEARCH AND THE POSITIVIST ATTITUDE

How does this contrast with the more usual roles and attitudes of positivist social science researchers? Sometimes the anthropological attitude is discussed in scholarly circles or reported in scientific papers, but usually it is not. As a result, many social scientists tend to be vague about the moral and interpersonal dimensions of their work. Unconsciously choosing a positivist theory of knowledge, they may believe that the most important goal in research is objectivity – being able to perceive, record, and analyze things the way they "really are." Often they fear that having close mutual relationships with research subjects will damage this objectivity in several ways: It might bring about change in the system under study, making it unique and therefore useless as an example. It also might cause the researcher's emotions to alter observation and analysis, another source of bias. Certainly, if the researcher admits a moral or emotional tie to the subjects, he fears his work will be taken less seriously by colleagues. And perhaps most important of all, the positivist believes that the choice of research questions and methods must be dictated not by the subjects of one's research, but by one's scientific peers and colleagues; that is, by the direction and traditions of one's discipline, about which the research subjects know nothing.

Given this set of attitudes, how is the traditional positivist researcher likely to feel and act in the research setting? Of course, researchers have personalities, and not everyone approaches his or her job in the same way. But on the whole, the positivist perspective encourages certain ways of thinking and working that differ from the anthropological attitude.

First, the traditional social researcher thinks of the research role as that of an expert on the subject of human behavior. By definition, this means that one should have a lot of knowledge about behavior that one's research subjects should not have. One should know a lot of specialized ideas (scientific theories) about why people behave as they do. One should know and use the specialized tools of social measurement to find out things about behavior that the people themselves do not know or understand. In contrast to the anthropological attitude, in which the research subjects are the experts and the researcher the student, this *expert* identity and role places the researcher in an elite position, a position that creates social distance between researcher and subject. Even if this social difference is never spoken of, it is expressed subtly in all the relationships between the studier and the studied.

To the traditional positivist researcher, this difference is natural and valuable. It simply reflects the true superiority of scientific knowledge over everyday knowledge and, after all, one's important and enduring social ties are with one's professional colleagues, not with one's research subjects. One hopes that the results of one's research will be helpful to the subject community, but that is secondary to the aim of advancing one's science, and of course one's career as a scientist. Such a researcher rarely expects the subject community to read or use the published results of the research. Lacking the scientific know-how – they are likely to lack the capacity to absorb, let alone use, the most important findings. Besides, sharing one's results with the subjects might influence their behavior, thereby changing the phenomena under study and ruining its experimental character.

In a related manner, the positivist researcher's focus on objectivity often leads to a mistrust of emotional engagement between researcher and subject. Of course there is a need to be polite with subjects, but the scientist must not become too involved. Interdependency should be kept to a minimum. This reinforces the first tendency, to maintain social distance between researcher and subject. The tendency in positivist research is to approach individual research subjects not as whole personalities with complex, patterned lives, but rather as cases, social units from whose lives the theoretically important variables (age, sex, health status, income, diet, certain attitudes, etc.) have been dissected and measured. One's emotional attitude toward a case is likely to be quite different than one's attitude toward a person.

A third, all-important, difference between the positivist and the anthropological approach to the research role has to do with *time* and *intensity*. Since the attempt is to achieve validity and reliability, the positivist seeks to develop measures that will yield the same results when applied by any trained researcher. The data must speak for themselves. Not only is it possible for the data collection and data analysis to be done independently, in some ways it is an ideal to be pursued. Moreover, once the research instruments have been properly refined, they should be applied in a straightforward, matter-of-fact way, with a minimum of interruption or conversation. Analysis will be well served if the data are standardized across people and situations. Too much variation in setting and process simply creates headaches for the analysts. All this means that the favored way to conduct positivist research is to field a team of trained researchers, gather the data quickly with streamlined, standardized instruments, and retire to the research office for the analysis. Besides, the quicker one gets results, the happier one's research sponsor and department chair will be, and the faster one will advance in one's career.

Contrast this picture with the slowness and intensity of the anthropological approach I have described. For the anthropologist, variations in individual perception and setting are critically important. Variations help to test and refine the researcher's evolving appreciation of patterns. Given broad constraints on time and energy, the deeper, more complex, and more unique a research encounter is, the better. In the example of the cockfight I gave at the beginning of this chapter, the arrival of the police was a stroke of luck for Geertz, because it helped deepen his understanding of the event.

The short term, low-intensity form of social research severely limits the kinds of data the positivist researcher can collect. Making the establishment of trust difficult, it may close off certain areas of thought and behavior from study. Seeking to standardize questions and observations makes it difficult to detect the ways in which setting (where, who, when, what activity, precursors and aftermath) and actors (status and power, role, age, gender, personality) affect perception and behavior. It severely limits the researcher's ability to observe gradually evolving situations of the sort that cannot be understood without the whole sequence. The positivist researcher's perspective is sometimes like that of someone who watches twenty minutes of a two-hour film, then tries to understand the plot.

Going back to the example of my relationship with Mrs. Kondo, imagine if I had simply appeared on her doorstep with an interview form one day, and had spent an hour or two giving standard questions before thanking her and disappearing from her life. Would I have learned about the nuances of social status in the new town, and gotten a hint of its real meaning for her?

We can clarify and summarize the differences between the anthropological and positivistic approaches to research with Table 4.1.

THE IMPORTANCE OF CONTEXTS IN SOCIAL RESEARCH

In Chapter Three, we discussed the important ability of the naturalistic theory of knowledge to help us deal with the problems of meaning and

Table 4.1 THE ANTHROPOLOGICAL AND POSITIVIST ROLES

	ANTHROPOLOGY	POSITIVISM
Theory of Knowledge	Naturalistic: Knowledge is the useful product of an interaction between interested observers and the observed.	Positivistic: Knowledge is an approximation of the actual state of a real world, verified by independent observers.
Main Research Strategy	Observe population in as many undisturbed natural settings as possible, in order to understand their point of view in context.	Use theory and hypotheses to posit relationships between variables extracted from population and measured precisely and objectively.
Objective	Understand perceived practical problems, thereby contributing to their solution.	Contribute to the advancement of objective knowledge, hopefully in a useful way.
Self and Role	Student, participant in group, seeking to learn from people who have superior knowledge of their world.	Expert, objective outsider, informed by accumulated knowledge of one's science.
Time and Intensity	Long-term total immersion in community, ideally for at least a year.	Selective, short-term, ideally a team of specialists using short, structured encounters over weeks or months.
Emotion	Emphasizes trust, with exchange of respect, obligation, sympathy.	Emphasizes objectivity, with control of research situation, minimal emotion.
Analysis	Proceeds concurrently with, and feeds continuously back to, data collection from start to finish.	Episodic, following waves of data collection.

context in human society. The significance of the anthropological attitude I have described in this chapter is that it allows us to apply this naturalistic way of observing and thinking. It allows us to observe normal behavior in settings that are as close as possible to the natural settings, or contexts, of everyday life. By demonstrating respect and openness at every opportunity, the researcher encourages people to feel that their ordinary way of talking and acting is appropriate and valuable, that there is no need to guard information or change things to make them more acceptable. We now return to the question of why it is so important to observe behavior this way.

As mentioned in Chapter Three, the basic principle that explains the importance of contexts in human life is that people's behavior is not guided simply by objective events, but rather by the *meaning* that people attach to those events. The meaning of events, in turn, is largely determined not by objective features of the events, but by customary rules of interpretation that vary from situation to situation. These rules are often ambiguous, and different actors may be applying different rules to a given situation, but the rules typically include questions about some of the following features:

1. In the repertoire of different kinds of familiar situations, what kind is this (work, sport, ritual, drama, humor, conflict, sexuality, crime, learning, etc.)?
2. Who are the main actors in this case (age, sex, social status, skills, reputation, etc.)?
3. How are they socially connected here (kin, neighbors, strangers, competitors, trading partners, teammates, superiors/inferiors, enemies, etc.)?
4. What led up to the situation (is it unique, customary, accidental, etc.), and what is expected to happen next (purpose of event, actors' motives, etc.)?

A good illustration of the application of interpretive rules is the way people – all people – use language. If I give you a common word, such as the word *love*, you will have a general idea of what it means, an idea that combines the many meanings of the word from its many different contexts. But notice how dramatically its meaning changes as we move from one context to another. Saying "John and Mary are in love" is somewhat different than "she loves her country." It is *very* different from "my dog loves to chase sticks," and even more different from, "is this love bird a male or a female?" or "the tennis game stands at three/love." Notice that the meaning of *love* is not a property of the word itself, but depends on the sentence in which it occurs. I can even make up new meanings for the word. Suppose I say, "Let's call the relationship between the notes in a harmonious musical chord *love*." If we agree to use the word that way, it has acquired yet a new meaning for us. You can play games like this with almost any common word. For purposes of this illustration, then, we can say that language entails the application of rules of interpretation to words-in-context.

All human social behavior works much the same way. As a simple example, what does it mean if someone looks directly at you and closes one eye? In American culture that can mean: (a) what I just said or did was a joke or a lie; (b) I find you sexually attractive; (c) we are both thinking something right now that we should not reveal; (d) I am skeptical about what you are saying; (e) or, it can have no social meaning – perhaps the person has an uncontrollable facial tick, or is merely practicing the gesture. The proper interpretation of the gesture must be found in the context in which it occurs. Of course, as with language, people make interpretive mistakes sometimes, and the result can cause a great deal of confusion. Other examples include the following:

- touching a person can be interpreted as (a) reassurance or affection, (b) threat or insult, (c) medical or other assistance, (d) sexual desire, (e) conveying information, (f) getting attention, (g) accident or clumsiness, (h) harmless curiosity;
- offering food can mean (a) fulfilling a duty or ritual role, (b) showing sympathy or friendship, (c) deflecting hostility, (d) exchange for equal worth, (e) seeking a favor, (f) showing honor or reverence;
- terms of address or epithets that are insulting between strangers ("boy" or "girl," "buddy," "fats," etc.) are often used to express affection between friends.

An important fact about the contextual nature of meaning is that most of the time people are not aware of the rules they are following, and therefore cannot explain them. Rarely does one meet people who can clarify the differences between contexts when asked. It is not unusual to meet people who *believe* they understand how a particular context affects a particular meaning, only to discover that the behavior in question does not fit their interpretations. All this means that most contextual meanings must be inferred from observed behavior. It is also risky to try to artificially re-create the context in question in order to study it, because it is difficult to know exactly what features of a given context are relevant to the choices of meaning that go with it.

Look again at the example of *Mrs. Ito*, in Chapter Three. Mrs. Ito was probably not aware that she was attaching a meaning to her situation that removed it from a class of situations we might call *interracial contact* and putting it in a class we might call, *being helped when sick*. Moreover, if I had tried to simulate the *being helped when sick* context in order to see how it affected racial interaction, I may well have created a situation that did not show the change I observed in the natural setting.

For a more complex example, look again at the example of *Ban Chan Village*, in Chapter Two. When the nurses circulated a questionnaire to measure the villagers' perceptions of local health problems, they created a *new context* for thinking about such issues. This new context had its own distinct actors, relationships, motives, and expectations. These features of the new situation were probably quite different from the natural ones that people were familiar with. We do not know how their answers to the questionnaire were affected by these features of the new context, but it would not be safe to assume that context and meaning were un-related. More important, as noted in Chapter Two, the questionnaire-giving context contained features that were not likely to elicit meanings that would be helpful either to the community or to the nurses. It pre-sented the nurses mainly as helpful but remote authority figures with unknown expectations, and the villagers mainly as passive sources of in-formation and victims of their own unhealthy lives – the exact opposite of the frame of mind that would be needed to produce optimistic and active cooperation between health workers and villagers toward a set of shared goals.

What did the anthropologically trained nurses do differently? The practice of anthropology as I have described it, over a period of many months in the village, prompted the following questions, which produced the kinds of information that suited the nurses' real problem: (In Chapter Five I discuss in detail how to develop a research problem.)

1. Are there any naturally occurring contexts in the village where people attribute to themselves and their neighbors such qualities as intelligence and skill, goodwill, and cooperativeness? If so what are these contexts?

2. If not, is there some natural process that could lead to the creation of a context like this?

3. What can be learned from other cooperative and competitive ac-tivities in the village about what encourages cooperation or com-petition? Have there been successful cooperative projects in the past, and if so how did they succeed?

4. Have there been attempts to mount cooperative projects in the village that failed, and if so, why did they fail?

5. How do people ordinarily resolve differences and build consensus?

6. What can be learned from their everyday behavior about how the villagers view the health workers? If necessary, how can this be changed?

7. Who in the village do they trust most, and least, and why?

8. What is their idea of *health*?

9. What priority do they place on health, as compared to other values such as social status, comfort, family values, and so forth?

10. What conflicts to they perceive among these various values? And finally,

11. Can the nurses help the villagers to participate in a natural context in which they might have productive discussions about whether,

and how, to improve the health of the village, and develop and carry out a plan for doing so?

12. What are the features (participants, time, place, type of activity, etc.) of this context, given what we have learned about meanings and contexts in this village?

SUMMARY

In the next two chapters, we examine further the art of asking anthropological questions. Here, let us summarize the main points of this chapter.

Anthropologists study human communities as integrated wholes, and this requires them to look closely at as many aspects of local behavior as possible. One of the objects in doing this is to understand the meanings people attach to their own behaviors and environments. This is necessary because humans rarely respond directly to their situations, but rather use culturally learned rules for attaching meaning to these situations, and use these meanings in designing their responses. The rules for *making meaning* differ from culture to culture, and from conventionally-defined situation to situation within a culture.

This point of view is of great importance to researchers who wish to help solve social problems. Such researchers must discover to some extent what things mean to the people in question, and how these meanings are made. They will benefit greatly from the anthropological way of observing people living their lives in as many of their natural settings as possible, so that the relationships between setting, meaning, and action can be understood. You can call anthropology the study of settings, or contexts. This way of working requires that the anthropologist take the role of a respectful student in the study community, and participate as openly and normally as possible in people's lives. This contrasts with the usual role of the positivist researcher. Positivists seek objectivity by controlling the data collection process as closely as possible, and minimizing the emotional element.

CHAPTER FIVE

Designing a Research Project

GUIDE TO THIS CHAPTER

In this chapter I outline the steps of developing a research project in anthropology. I do not claim that this is the only way to do anthropological research, or that it is a complete guide to solving every kind of research problem. Instead, I introduce the student to a set of basic steps that explains how to select a problem and begin to work on the answer. These steps apply to every kind of practical research problem in anthropology, and they help researchers make good decisions about what to study and how to study it, and to avoid many common mistakes made by health workers who wish to use an anthropological point of view.

The main points made in this chapter are as follows:

1. Following the naturalistic theory of knowledge, all anthropological research seeks to find useful answers to problems (see Chapter Three for a definition of *useful*).
2. The research process begins with a partial, incomplete understanding of the things we want to know at the end of the study, and a clear idea of our purpose, that is, why we want to know this. Together, we call this partial understanding and the purpose of the work *intuition* (see Chapter Three).
3. The research project makes the intuition more clear, complete, and useful by following three steps. These steps are taken not once, but many times, and not in a fixed order, but constantly going back and forth according to what needs to be done next. The three steps are:
    i. making each part of the intuition as clear as possible;
    ii. looking at cases that illustrate parts of the intuition, to see if the parts and the relationships fit; and
    iii. revising and improving the whole intuition, bit by bit, so that it is more complete and useful, and so that it fits the actual situation we are observing better.

4. Because one is looking for useful answers to specific questions, and not trying to discover universal *truth*, it is extremely important to be clear about the study questions, and why and how one is asking those particular questions. Good questions are those that:
   i. answer practical problems, as determined by our values as researchers;
   ii. can be studied using the resources (skills, time, money) we have at hand;
   iii. produce results that persuade others (community, co-workers, government) that the research is useful.

One of the first things you will notice about this method is that it is not linear, it does not follow a straight line from A to B to C, the way much quasi-laboratory research does. Rather, it is a circular process, in which the researcher repeatedly goes back to earlier steps and revises them. One way to think about this is to imagine you are putting together the pieces of a picture puzzle, without knowing what the final picture is supposed to look like. You will make guesses about where each piece goes, often many times, before you find its correct place. You might also form theories about what the final picture will look like, and you will have to revise these theories as you discover the true relationships among the pieces. But don't forget, with this puzzle, there may be more than one *correct* picture!

THE PROCESS OF DETAILED UNDERSTANDING

About 2,500 years ago, the Greek philosopher Plato made an interesting observation: If you want to have a precise, detailed understanding of something, you cannot start from complete ignorance. To understand it more clearly, you must already know quite a bit about what you want to study in order to know where to begin. For example, suppose you want to know the exact definition of *health*. Where will you start? You can start by comparing people who are *healthy* with people who are not, to see what the similarities and differences are. But how do you know who is healthy or not, unless you already know what health is? Well, you can start with a definition of health, and then see who fits it and who does not. But that does not solve the puzzle. What good is the definition, unless we can imagine whom it fits and whom it does not fit? Actually, in order to ask the question, we must know something about both the definition of health, and its real expression in the world.

This is true of all detailed understanding. We can describe the basic process by which anything is clearly and thoroughly known (including all scientific knowledge) as follows:

1. There are three parts to the process of detailed understanding:
   a. intuition of the whole,
   b. specification of parts, and
   c. comparison of cases.
2. These three parts of the process are mutually interdependent. None of them can proceed far without the others. They are like the three legs of a stool. Without any one of the legs, the stool will not stand.
3. One must begin with an *intuition* of the whole. This intuition specifies some of the parts of the thing to be understood, and some of the relationships among these parts, but it is not yet detailed or clear. This intuition tells one what might constitute a case, and what some of the parts might be.
4. From the intuited configuration, one can move either to the identification of cases, or to the further specification of parts. The former is called the inductive method, and the latter is called the deductive method.
5. One moves back and forth from each process to the others repeatedly, using the *intuition* to guide the discovery of cases and the identification of parts, the *cases* to test the validity of the evolving intuition, and the *parts* to discover or reject and examine more cases, and refine and develop the intuition into a detailed understanding.
6. This process has no ideal end-state. It continues until one either runs out of time to pursue it, or decides that one's understanding is detailed enough.

This process can be diagrammed as seen in Figure 5.1.

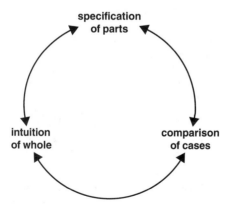

Figure 5.1   The process of detailed understanding.

EXAMPLE: The Detailed Understanding Process: What Does My Community Mean by "Alcoholism?"

In giving an example of the process of detailed understanding, I want to simply add concrete imagery to the process so that it will be easier to imagine. I want to avoid examples that are very complicated, even though they may be more interesting to health workers. So I will choose a fairly simple definition problem. Imagine you are a community health worker, and many people say they are concerned about alcoholism in the community. You are not sure you understand what they mean.

Your intuition about what alcoholism is tells you that alcoholism might be an important health concern, and you should know more about what they mean. People who cause problems because of the effects of drinking beer, whiskey, wine, and so on are usually called alcoholics. The problems usually have something to do with the impairment of judgment and performance that affects people who drink too much.

You begin to specify the parts of your intuition: Some people who drink alcohol, even quite a lot, may not be called alcoholics, if they do not cause trouble for themselves or others. Some people might be suspected of drinking secretly if they behave like they are drunk, but might actually have some other problem, such as drug use or mental illness. Drunkenness might be considered a shame by the families of those called alcoholics, because it might be associated with moral failure. Alcoholics might cause fear and even physical injury to themselves or others, and they might waste resources that could be used for family health and well-being. This is the beginning of a list of parts of your intuition about alcoholism, and you can add your own ideas.

This list of parts gives you a list of questions to ask people about what alcoholism is. What kinds of things do people believe alcoholics do? When and where? Who else is involved? How do they get drunk? Who objects to their behavior, and why? Is there such a thing as drinking "reasonably," and what is that? Are there "okay" and "bad" alcoholics?" What makes the difference? Your list of questions should examine each of the important parts of your intuition.

As you begin to ask these questions, you also begin to collect cases. You ask people to identify some of the alcoholics, and talk about what these specific people are like, and why they are considered alcoholics. You also ask about people who drink alcohol but are not alcoholics, people who cause problems but do not drink, and so on. You note differences of opinion about the matter. You make a point of observing the people who are discussed, to see how your observation fits or does not fit with what others say.

The cases lead you to specify more parts, to refine your intuition. Let us suppose you discover that people who regularly get drunk and unruly during festivals are not considered alcoholics, but those who do so at other times and places – for example at home or during solemn rituals – are. Also, certain kinds of potentially dangerous behavior while drunk, such as working with dangerous tools, swimming, or driving, are not considered alcoholism, while other kinds, such as fighting or wife beating, are.

Suppose you discover that people who beat their wives or fight are often suspected of drinking too much, even when there is no other evidence that they do so. Also, perhaps influential people can behave in a disorderly way while drunk without being identified as alcoholics, while humble people cannot, and women are much more likely to get the label if they drink than men. Perhaps in this community, drinking alcohol in itself is not considered particularly dangerous to the drinker's health. Certain religious groups might be considered more sober than others, even though statistically this does not appear true.

Suppose in this community alcohol is readily available illegally, in spite of official efforts to control it. People who are not considered alcoholics are just as likely to buy it illegally as those who are. This would indicate that many people value it highly, and it may be difficult to reduce its general use much. Those who sell alcohol in the community, and their friends and families, might tend to deny that drinking is a serious problem here.

In addition to your interviews and observations in this community, there are other sources of cases and parts. You can go to the nearby college library and read what you can find about: (1) the history, folklore, and customs having to do with alcohol in this region; (2) local laws about alcohol use; (3) health, illness, medicine, and alcohol use, both in general and in this region; (4) the portrayal of alcohol in advertising, films, TV, and popular music.

Now you can refine your intuition about what alcoholism means. In this community, it is a label that applies to certain very specific kinds of disruptive behavior, which might or might not actually involve the use of alcohol. Much behavior that you consider hazardous is not defined as alcoholism. There is a gender and a class bias to the label, women and poor people being more susceptible to it. You might add the intuition that social attitudes, personal profit, and ideas about alcoholism are closely related. Methods of marketing alcohol may have become very sophisticated, and young people may be more likely now to abuse it than in years past.

Now you have a much more detailed and accurate idea of what people mean when they complain about alcoholism, and this knowledge is very useful. If you want to help the community address it, you might think about either teaching them about the unrecognized problems drinking causes, or helping them focus the issue of interpersonal violence from all causes, if that seems to be their real concern.

If you are really interested in this issue, you can continue to refine your intuition about it, trying to discover how personal background and experience leads to drinking or sobriety, why some drinkers are more violent than others, which methods of preventing alcoholism seem to work in this context and which do not, and so on. You might even want to begin to develop a theory of alcoholism that will fit this community and others like it better than existing theories.

IDENTIFYING A RESEARCH PROBLEM

The most important, and often the most difficult, part of doing anthro-pological research on health is the proper identification of a problem to study. Our ideas about what we want to know will greatly influence how we see everything about the community we are studying. We must struggle constantly to remain open to the question of whether we are asking the right questions – questions that will produce useful answers. In order to do this, we must clearly determine two things: (1) why we have chosen this problem, and (2) how we will recognize the answer.

Why Have We Chosen This Problem?

This question forms an important part of the original *intuition* that begins the research, and is in itself complex. It includes at least the following complex sub-questions:

1. What are our *ethical priorities* in doing this research? What do we care most about in a moral sense? Improving the average person's enjoyment of life? Relieving the suffering of the sickest? Correcting inequalities in access to resources? Strengthening human dignity by improving the autonomy and self-respect of the group? Other values? If our priorities include all of these factors, might there be conflicts among them – and if so, which is the most important? A clash between our values and those of the people we want to study might destroy any good we hope to achieve – are we in harmony?

2. What *theories* or models of health and social behavior are relevant to these priorities? In other words, what aspects of behavior and situation do we need to understand in order to work toward our values, and why? For example, what has the most effect on people's health and happiness, their cultural health beliefs, their access to resources, or their self-respect? What processes lead most surely to lasting change in any one of these areas? In Chapters Nine and Ten of this book, I propose models of *health behavior* and *community empowerment* that suggest specific relationships between: (a) values, such as equality and dignity; (b) health; and, (c) research methods.

3. What do we *already know about this setting* that can guide us to a practical sense of the problem. What are the needs and priorities of the people in the setting? What sources of data are likely to be the most accurate and available? Does the problem we have selected make sense, given our local knowledge? Will members of the community themselves be able to join in action to solve the problem?

4. What *research methods* best support our ethical priorities and at the same time lead to effective answers? Can we select methods that contribute to the dignity and equality of the people we study, while at the same time encouraging them to reflect critically on their way of life? Can we serve our values by strengthening

relationships between the researchers and their respondents through the research process? Are there kinds of questions that can be effectively addressed by ethically excellent research methods, and kinds that cannot?

How Will We Recognize the Answer?

This simple-looking question, which must also be part of the starting point of intuition, holds the key to the value of scientific research of all kinds. Very often it is not carefully studied during the design of a research project, and the result is a set of final information that does not do much to solve the main research problem. Go back to the example of *Ban Chan Village*, at the beginning of Chapter Two. The researchers wanted to strengthen the ability of the health care system to serve the needs of the village. They hoped to do this by studying the people's perceptions of the problems, and then designing interventions that met people's needs. At first, they decided that the answers to a questionnaire about village problems would lead them to the answer to their research question. However, this led to serious problems. They thought they were looking for objective facts that had little to do with their relationship with the villagers, or the villagers' relationships with each other. Accordingly:

- they used a method that reinforced the social distance between the villagers (passive, needing help, uninformed) and the health workers (active, empowered, expert);
- they did not consider how they would use the results of their survey to produce practical solutions;
- they did not have a useful theory or model about the relationships between the questionnaire results and their original intentions. Such a model would have tried to specify at least (1) how local perceptions of problems are formed and changed; (2) the relationship between perceptions of problems on one hand, and feelings of effectiveness, or ability to take action, on the other; (3) how the local health system and other stake-holders (for example, elites) helped to shape perceptions.

When the researchers thought carefully about what the answer to their question would look like, they chose to approach it from a different angle. They became participants in the village instead of outside *experts*, and they offered, first, to help the villagers think for themselves about ways to improve their lives. Then the researchers aided them in crafting creative solutions to things that the villagers themselves felt they might be able to change. The result was a subtle change in the way some villagers thought about *problems*, and, eventually, a highly useful answer to the question, "How can we work with the villagers to improve their health?"

In order to be able to work toward the solution of any research problem, it is essential that we researchers constantly question the value of all results in the light of our original purpose, and *be ready to change the project* either to get different results, or to explore new areas suggested by incoming data. In some cases, one might find that the original research problem was flawed, as it did not really suit the values of the researcher. In most research, the original intuition contains errors and blind leads, and these must be discovered and eliminated. *Only by having a clear sense of purpose can we recognize whether a particular observation really contributes toward the answer, and make the necessary changes if it does not.*

This might be a bit difficult to understand right now, but it will become clearer as we discuss the next steps – formulating questions and analyzing data.

The Problem Statement

Sometimes research problems are developed originally from abstract knowledge about a community. We might have data showing high rates of diabetes and heart disease, and want to know what cultural and environmental factors are contributing to these in a particular population; or we might find that many people are using a certain kind of native healer, and want to know why this is the case, and what the effects are on overall population health.

Sometimes, problem statements grow naturally out of our daily observation of life in the community. In talking to people about health, for example, we might discover that many people are troubled about something that we had not recognized at first and know little about. In the midst of observing other things, we begin to develop a problem statement that will allow us to understand this new one.

For example, in my work on health in low-income neighborhoods in Alameda County, among the things I discovered were: First, teenage girls seemed to be less happy than boys or older people in general. Second, these girls often talked about feeling pressured to have sex. To my list of research tasks, I felt it was important to add the problem: How do sexual attitudes and behavior contribute to stress for these girls, with what results?

Whether our sense of the problem arises from abstract statistical information or from our daily experience in the community, it is useful to

have a systematic statement of the problem that contains all the elements
I have identified: our purpose for engaging in the research to begin with
(values, sense of need, desired outcome), our theoretical ideas about the
problem, our knowledge of the research setting, and the methods we think
we can use to get answers.

Continuing with the example of sexual harassment and stress, I might
formulate the problem as follows:

- *Values and goals*: I believe people of all income levels and back-
  grounds should have equal opportunities for health and well-
  being. If their circumstances limit their opportunities, I would like
  to contribute to changing this situation. I also believe that research,
  like any other social activity, should support the values of human
  equality, freedom, and dignity, and that therefore I should consider and conduct myself as an equal with those I study. I should
  consider their culture, beliefs and opinions, and goals as equal in
  value to mine.
- *Outcome*: I would like the members of this community to have a
  better understanding of the conditions that affect their health and
  well-being, and of the actions they might take to improve things.
  I believe communities of all kinds have the ability to understand
  their own problems and develop solutions to them.
- *Background knowledge*: I have very little knowledge of the issue I am about to study. I do not know whether my data about
  stress in adolescent women or its causes are correct or not. I do
  know that many older residents of this neighborhood are worried about the stress affecting young people and about their behavior, including the use of drugs and alcohol, and sex. I have
  read many ethnographic studies of low-income neighborhoods
  with some similarities to this one. Several of these studies discuss sources of stress for low-income families, men, children, and
  women. I have studied the recent history of this community with
  respect to housing, employment, migration, and ethnicity. I participate in monthly meetings on health problems with several of the
  residents.
- *Theories and models*: As a theory of knowledge, I follow the naturalistic theory. Among the theoretical models I find useful are the
  five needs model (see Chapter Nine) and the *theory of hope* (see
  Chapter Ten).
- *Methods*: In keeping with the naturalistic theory of knowledge and
  the values that inform this study, I use participant observation and
  informal interviewing, usually face to face. I believe the best results

are obtained when the researcher, as a peer, shares his observations freely with members of the community under study.

The Intuition Statement

Since exact knowledge is gained by refining one's original intuition, it is important to make this intuition as clear as possible at the beginning of the research, and to keep a record of it, so that you will be able to reconstruct just how it changed, and what data were used to improve it. Early on in the work, you should write an *intuition statement*. This statement should be preserved and reviewed periodically during the research, and new statements written which show how and why it changed in the light of data. Each intuition statement should include answers to the following questions:

- What do all your previous observations, reports, and related experience suggest to you about your research problem?
- What theories or models might help to understand it?
- What knowledge is missing from your intuition, and how might you look for that knowledge?

Note, again, that the purpose of your study is not to "prove" that your intuition is correct! The purpose is to improve the intuition by making it fit the problem and the data more closely, and become richer, more complex, and more practical.

EXAMPLE: How to Formulate an Intuition Statement: "What Does My Community Mean by 'Alcoholism'?"

1. *What is usually meant by alcoholism? Usually the word refers not just to people who drink alcoholic beverages, including wine, beer, whisky, and mixtures of these things with other beverages, like coke and fruit juice. Usually it refers to people whose behavior is viewed by their community or family as a "problem," that is caused by their drinking itself.*
2. *What are the different kinds of alcoholism? In some places, there are those who drink continuously, and there are others who alternate between periods of sobriety and drunkenness. There are those who only become slightly impaired due to drinking, and there are those who drink to the point of unconsciousness or serious illness. Different age groups and sexes may have different alcoholism characteristics. Teenagers, young adults, and the elderly might be viewed differently, as men and women might be.*
3. *What kinds of problem behavior occur with alcoholism? Usually, there can be several kinds of alcoholic behavior: (a) alcoholics might become too emotional (sad, talkative, angry), so that they cause problems for others,*

sometimes including violence; (b) they might forget to do important things that others need them to do; (c) they might not be able to work, so that they become a burden or a shame to their family or community; (d) they may just behave in a stupid or impolite way, so that people around them are embarrassed; (e) they might spend too much money on alcohol, or on other unnecessary things when they are drunk; (f) they might accidentally hurt themselves or other people when they are drunk.

4. What kinds of drinking behavior are not alcoholism? Usually, drinking alcohol is not called "alcoholism" if: (a) it is part of a ritual, or is expected to occur under normal circumstances, such as at parties or ceremonies, or in certain places, such as a men's club; (b) people who drink do not become "drunk" in the sense of changing their behavior too much; (c) it is part of a social role, for example, a shaman drinking in order to achieve insight into an illness; (d) it is done only to relieve temporary physical or mental suffering, such as an injury or an emotional trauma; (e) the person who becomes drunk does so only rarely, not as a habit.

5. How does alcoholism affect other people, and why are they concerned about it? Concern over alcoholism is probably related to the specific relationship between the alcoholic and the concerned person. A family member might be concerned because the alcoholic behavior is either embarrassing, or dangerous, or damaging to other family members' health or emotional state, or financially damaging to the family. A neighbor might be concerned because the alcoholic embarrasses the community, or inflicts displeasure by rude behavior, or threatens harm by clumsiness or aggression.

6. What is the moral dimension of alcoholism? It could be a moral failure of the alcoholic or his family, or a natural or supernatural, mental, or physical illness. Illness itself might be morally neutral, or might result from the evil of either the victim or someone else.

7. What is appropriate behavior toward alcoholics and their families? Depending on the drinker's characteristics (status, role, age and gender, drinking behavior), and the explanation of the behavior, they and their families might be shunned, treated by a specialist, ignored, punished, held in contempt, or given special status.

8. What other social factors might be important in shaping the problem? (a) It stands to reason that relationships of power would be an important factor. Probably, the more power the alcoholic person A has over person B, the more concerned B will be about A's behavior. (b) Cultural explanations of drinking in general, and of alcoholism in particular, will play an important role. Why do people drink? How does alcohol affect a person? Who is able to drink wisely, and who is not, and why? (c) Attitudes of outsiders might also be important, especially attitudes of health workers, teachers, government officials, and religious figures – people whose opinions are important in the community. (d) There may be specialists, such as shamans who treat alcohol-related problems, and they might have a distinct view of what it is, what causes it, and how to treat it.

Notice several things about this intuition statement:

1. It is *incomplete*. It does not try to tell you everything you need to know about the community's definition of alcoholism. It is meant only to give you a starting place.
2. It is based on what you already *know* about alcoholism, just from what you have seen and heard before doing the research; in other words, it is a set of *untested suppositions*, which your research will test and modify.
3. There is no *universal formula* or outline for your intuition. Simply state what you think is important based on your pre-existing knowledge, and state it in a way that feels systematic and makes sense to you.
4. It helps you decide *what to observe* (cases and parts). For example, you need to look for alcoholism in which the *status or power* of the drinker varies; you need to talk to people who are *relatives* and *nonrelatives* of the drinker; you need to observe and ask about male, female, young and old drinkers; you need to interview laymen and specialists (cases). You need to ask what is *problematic* about the drinking in question and why, why some people drink too much and others don't, who drinks but is not "alcoholic," and so on (parts).
5. It is thoroughly *practical*. It focuses on dimensions of alcoholism that you can reasonably observe and ask about, and it deals with the practical dimensions of the problem – the impact it might have on people's well- being. It avoids such abstract issues as whether alcoholism is *really* an "illness" or a "sin."
6. As you collect data on the question, you will keep coming back to this statement and performing two tasks: First, you will make changes and add refinements based on what you are learning. Second, you will look for questions that still remain unanswered, which will guide your next research steps.

Now we return to the formulation of specific research questions.

FORMULATING SPECIFIC RESEARCH QUESTIONS

Because the answers to anthropological research questions often change our perception of what we are studying, it is difficult to design a research problem that will turn out to produce the results we originally imagined. Remember Plato's discovery: In order to know something precisely, we have to begin by knowing it in a general way. Our first try at formulating a research problem is based on our general knowledge of the situation, what I have called the *intuition*, which might have big inaccuracies and gaps in it. We should expect to keep looking at our problem statement to see if it continues to make sense in the light of our two guiding principles: (1) the usefulness of the envisioned answer (see Chapter Three), and (2) our emerging findings. What often happens is that we gradually find out that some of the questions we are asking do not produce useful information, and we must consider other questions. Sometimes we discover that either what we originally considered a desirable outcome is impossible, or that some other outcome would actually be more desirable.

EXAMPLE: *Thai Subjects Find the Research Question Irrelevant*

A friend of mine was studying the way people grow old in different cultures. He was especially interested in what kind of social relationships people have later in life, and how this affects their health and well-being. After reading a good deal about Southeast Asian cultures, his intuition was that Thailand would make a nice contrast to America, so he learned Thai and went there. As he interviewed aged Thais about their lives, he became more and more frustrated. Although most of them had close friends and family, almost no one was at all interested in his topic of social relations. No matter what he asked them about it, they would change the subject. Usually what they really wanted to talk about was death and afterlife. After trying for weeks to get them back onto his subject, it suddenly struck him: If he wanted to understand aging in Thailand, he was asking entirely the wrong questions. The health and well-being of the elderly depended less on the details of their social interactions than on the depth of their religious faith, and their sense of spiritual security. He ended up focusing on the different ways in which Thais and Americans understand and deal with death. With this information in the foreground, many important differences in their social relationships, and the effects of relationships on mental health, became clear to him.

So we do the best we can to formulate a good statement of the problem, one that takes into account our values, our theories, the methods we might use, and our need for answers. Next, we examine the knowledge we already have about the problem, and ask ourselves, "What is missing, if we are going to find useful answers to the problem, using the methods and situation at hand?" This leads us to the next steps in clarifying the problem: "What is already known about it that I can easily get access to?" And, "within the easily available information, what are the obvious gaps?"

At this stage, theories or models are often quite helpful. By a *theory*, I mean a fairly complete and well-developed idea that other scholars have

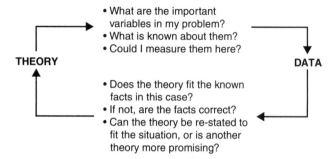

Figure 5.2   Relationship between theory and data.

used to explain a social phenomenon. Using the example above, my friend was interested in trying to apply a theory called "disengagement," which holds basically that as people age, they lose energy and interest in social relationships, and begin to give them up or put less emphasis on them.

By a *model*, I mean a less complete or well-developed idea about how things are related. For example, if people will not cooperate with health authorities even to do something simple that would help their health, the *local interest* model suggests that these people are more concerned about other problems, and that one must meet these concerns first if one wants them to cooperate. As mentioned in Chapter Three, theories and models specify the relationships among facts, and by trying to apply a potentially useful theory or model to our own research question, we can see more clearly what facts are missing. At the same time, by looking at the facts we do have, we can begin to judge what theories might be useful. We can diagram the relationship as seen in Figure 5.2.

It is helpful to pursue this process of question formulation very, very thoroughly, and to consider any and all reasonable models that seem to fit the available knowledge and to promise useful solutions. For this purpose, it is useful to know about a wide variety of theories and models having to do with the area of behavior in which one is interested, in order to consider the many ways of forming the research question and the many kinds of observations that might contribute to the solution of the problem. Again, going back to *Ban Chan Village*, the nurses in that example considered mainly the local interest model of social change. To this they might have added other models and theories, such as the following:

- *cultural strain*, the idea that social problems arise when techno-logical change is too rapid, so that habitual solutions to social problems no longer work;

- *hierarchy of needs* (see Chapter Nine), the idea that solutions to human problems must meet a certain basic list of human needs; and,
- *socially desirable response set*, that if you ask people for an opinion they will give you one, even if they have never considered the question and have no interest in the answer.

Characteristics of Good Questions

Once we have achieved clarity of purpose, have the best intuition we can manage about what we are seeking, and have learned what we can both from theory and background data about our study population, what principles can guide us in forming useful questions?

We must have reason to believe that the questions we ask *will produce answers that are useful* in solving our research problem. This means we must have some confidence that the answers we get are not arbitrary or random with respect to our problem – the naturalistic equivalent of relevance, validity, and reliability. This is exactly why we must begin with an intuition of what the parts of the problem are.

Many, but not all, good questions can be answered by several *different kinds of data*, in case one type is misleading. For example, if we want to know what people mean by "alcoholism," we can learn by asking questions, by watching behavior, listening to casual conversation, and studying literature, drama, and so on.

Good questions *lend themselves to study* in the situation at hand. I might not be able to answer a questionsuch as, "What are the main causes of suffering in this community?" because the sources of unhappiness might be too private, too idiosyncratic, and too hard to describe or explain. I might be able to ask questions about clinical depression, because I could administer clinical tests for depression. But I must be sure that the data that result *will actually contribute to the answer to my research problem*. If I am really interested in subjective unhappiness, and not clinical diagnoses, the clinical data might not be helpful in itself.

Good questions are general enough that we will not miss important information. If I suspect that sexual harassment is an important source of stress for teenage girls in my community, I should ask not just about sexual harassment alone, I should also ask about other sources of stress and things that relieve stress, and about the characteristics of people and situations that make a sexual experience stressful or not.

Good questions are specific enough that they will allow me to assess the relevance of the answers to the research problem. Staying with the example of sexual harassment and stress, I would want to know all the various meanings people attach to "stress" and "sexual harassment," and whether their meanings fit with my intuition.

Good questions focus on important comparisons suggested by our intuition. If our intuition says that stress, age, and gender are important factors (again the example of sexual pressure is a good one), we should try to compare similar situations where age and gender vary. First, we might look at girls who are extremely stressed by such pressures, and those who are not, to see what other factors might be involved. Next, we might look at sources of stress among older women and young men, to see what their sources of stress are, and how they handle it.

RESEARCH DESIGN AS A CONTINUOUS PROCESS

It should now be clear that the formation of a research problem and the development of questions are the first steps in the research process, but they are steps that are never finished until the research is complete. The research problem, based on one's intuition of the whole, suggests what questions to ask – the specification of parts – and these in turn suggest what methods to use and what and whom to observe – the comparison of cases. In the next two chapters we examine the process of actually collecting data; but we must keep in mind that the process of design that we have been discussing in this chapter continues throughout the research process. As new observations are made and new analyses done, the researcher continuously revisits and reformulates the basic problem, the intuition behind it, and the original questions. This, of course, is the natural way in which most human work gets done.

SUMMARY

The steps in designing an anthropological research project do not follow a linear sequence; rather, they are processes that the researcher revisits over and over again, working toward clarity and persuasiveness. The steps always include the following:

- Defining the research problem. This includes being clear about why you selected this problem, and how you plan to study it. This should be stated in a written *problem statement* of the kind given on pages 79–80.
- Clarifying your intuition about the problem. What do you already know about it, and what do you not know that you need to? You

should write an *intuition statement* early in the research process, and keep a record of how it changes during the process, and why.

- Selecting cases that illustrate your intuition.
- Comparing the actual data from the cases with your intuition, and clarifying the intuition by specifying its details.

We discussed the criteria for good research problems, and for good questions to ask in order to clarify them.

CHAPTER SIX

The Researcher in and Beyond the Community

GUIDE TO THIS CHAPTER

In this chapter, we will consider in detail the relationship between the anthropologist and the community he or she studies. The most important skill that a health anthropologist must learn is to secure the strong trust and cooperation of the people he or she is studying. Without this trust and cooperation, the value of one's research is questionable, and one's ability to use the results to improve people's lives is doubtful.

I have already mentioned that the traditional social science roles of the *outside expert* or *neutral observer* are neither necessary nor desirable in doing naturalistic social science. Rather, the anthropologist seeks to get close to the study community, to accept and be accepted in the ways people naturally relate to each other in everyday life. The questions that face us here, then, are as follows:

1. What kinds of tasks are required of a naturalistic social scientist, and what type of behavior in the study setting is best suited to those tasks?
2. What notions of truth and justice best support naturalistic social science, and how do those notions bear on the behavior of the researcher?
3. How should the research process be affected by the researcher's relationships with (a) scientific colleagues and (b) society at large?

PARTICIPANT OBSERVATION

In Chapters Two though Five, we discussed how the naturalistic social scientist seeks to understand communities in a way that is useful in the context of their local and present way of life. I mentioned that, in order to do this, the researcher avoids taking bits of behavior, or *variables*, out of their local situation and using them to test abstract models of behavior.

Rather, it is precisely the interrelationships of things – health, work, play, money, religion, learning, morals, sex, family life, art, history – that one tries to grasp. I often say to my students that *anthropology is the study of contexts*. In Chapter Three I discussed, for example, the way context affects meaning, and meaning affects behavior, in such a manner that we can understand behavior best if we study it in its natural situations. In Chapter Eleven, we will revisit the role of the researcher in the context of *action anthropology*.

Let me reintroduce the process of *participant observation* I discussed in Chapter Three. The best way to preserve contextual relationships is to observe, (first-hand whenever possible) how all these things are in fact related in the way people live their everyday lives. Although the logistics of research often require us to modify the ideal of participant observation, that ideal is that the researcher:

- lives among the people being studied, in a setting similar to the way they live (housing, food, dress, etc.), for several months or years at a time;
- masters and uses the local language and customs reasonably well, to minimize the awkwardness of his or her presence;
- participates as an equal in the collective activities of life – group work, recreation, rituals and celebrations, meetings, and just "hanging around";
- shares his or her own resources (food, transportation, skills, advice, etc.) with the community according to custom.

The advantages of this way of working, if it is done properly, are great:

1. The researcher gradually ceases to be a curiosity or a disruption in community life. Life can then proceed more or less normally, which gives validity to the researcher's observations.
2. Most people lose the natural suspicion they have of strangers when interacting with the participant observer. A level of trust grows that encourages people to speak the truth and to reveal things they would not tell a stranger, or perhaps even a neighbor (see the example of *Mrs. Kondo* in Chapter Four).
3. Being in the community during all hours of the day and night, all days of the week and month, and all seasons of the year gives the researcher an opportunity to see many of the cyclical variations that form part of ordinary life – work, leisure, rituals, seasonal activities, and so on. With luck, the researcher can observe the great life events as well – birth, coming of age, marriage, retirement, and death.

4. Learning the personalities of community members, and the details of their relationships with each other, allows the researcher to avoid certain conflicts and build certain alliances to make his or her work easier.

5. In cases where the researcher has special knowledge to contribute to community life, such as health knowledge for example, participant observation may improve the chance that such knowledge can be shared and used by the community.

ETHICS AND VALUES

The advantages of participant observation, however, demand a price. Before we turn to the practical discussion of the most effective roles and attitudes for doing this kind of work, we need to talk about its ethical burdens. Taking part in people's lives is a morally sensitive thing to do for several reasons. First, the researcher is usually better educated and may have more social status and a higher income than most of the people being studied. This creates an imbalance in power; it gives the researcher more knowledge, security, and opportunities than the others. In such a situation, it is often too easy for the researcher to take advantage of people, or to be insensitive to their needs.

The researcher is also asking local people to reveal details of their lives, but usually does not reveal his/her own life the same way. This contributes to the gap in power. It also requires great care to protect people's safety, privacy, and dignity, both within the local community, and in the world at large. Moreover, the researcher is usually only a temporary visitor in the community. He or she will soon leave, and unlike others, will not have to deal with ongoing problems there. Keeping in mind the long-term implications of what one sees, and especially of one's own actions, is both difficult and important.

The researcher often provides to the wider society a picture of what the community is like, a picture that can be used either to the advantage or the disadvantage of the residents. One must try to be aware of the possible uses of what one reports.

For all these reasons, simple decency requires strict rules about the ethics of doing participant observation, even when the researcher is not required by law or contract to follow these rules. The minimum rules are as follows:

1. *Openness and honesty about oneself.* The researcher may never conceal her identity or general purpose from the researched. On the contrary, she must make sure that people who are studied

clearly know who she is, why she is there, who supports her research, and what she expects to do with the results of the study. This is limited only by rule two, confidentiality. Changes in the methods or goals of the study must be discussed with participants. Care should be taken that people also know the limits of the researcher's abilities, knowledge, and resources.

2. *Confidentiality about others.* The researcher must always behave in such a way that information gotten in private remains private, and that the names and identities of participants are kept secret wherever possible. The only exception is when specific permission to share information is freely given by the participants. It is best not to discuss within the community things that happen in public either, unless there is a good reason to do so. This rule applies not just to notes from conversations and observations, but to data from records, photographs, maps, and other kinds of records.

3. *Respect for beliefs, values, and feelings.* Being invited into a community to take part in people's lives and learn their thoughts is a great privilege and honor. But the greater the cultural and social class differences between the researcher and the researched, the more difficult it is to feel and show respect for everything about the people one is working among. This respect is extremely important, because it forms the background attitude that finally determines how we relate to people, and what we do with the information they give us. Respect is an indispensable ingredient of productive human relations. The absence of respect in itself breeds conflict and suffering. This does not mean that the researcher should tolerate behavior that local people do not tolerate among themselves, such as violence, gross irresponsibility, or theft. It also does not mean agreeing with the wisdom or justness of everything others do.

Ethics for Other Styles of Research

Participant observation is almost always one of the methods an anthropologist uses in community research. Often the situation does not permit the ideal of local long-term residence and active engagement in the full round of community life. Anthropologists increasingly study commuter towns, factory workers, clinic patients, or professional groups whose lives are simply not visible continuously or in one place. Anthropologists might be called on to study several communities simultaneously, to lead teams of interviewers, or to include survey techniques among their methods. In such cases, what ethical principles should apply? In my view, the basic rules I have described should apply to anthropological research using any methodology.

In addition to these minimum rules, the researcher's institution might require a set of formal procedures, usually overseen by an *institutional review board (IRB)*, specifying how the rights and safety of research subjects are to be protected. These rules vary from place to place, and I will not explore them in this book.

Observing Unacceptable Behavior

The activity of trying to understand how other people view the world usually leads to sympathy with their way of living and thinking. But occasionally anthropologists observe things that are so different from their own ideas of right and wrong that they are shocked or outraged. Many Westerners are appalled by the Middle Eastern religious practice of mutilating female genitals, or the Hindu custom of forcing a man's widow to join his funeral pyre. Some very dangerous folk medical practices, such as smearing dung on a newborn's umbilicus, shock health workers. Ethnographers sometimes witness serious illegal behaviors, too, such as drug dealing, financial cheating, political graft, or theft.

What is the researcher to do when an observed behavior seems outrageous and intolerable?

Should one try to convince those involved to stop the practice? Try to get the legal system or local power structure to stop it? Ignore one's own feelings and simply tolerate it? Pack up and abandon the research project? Publish articles condemning it?

Anthropologists call this dilemma the *problem of cultural relativity* – should we consider all behaviors accepted by the group under study to be morally acceptable, or should we insist that there are universal moral laws, and that violations of these laws are acts against nature? There is no generally accepted solution to the cultural relativity question.

In my view, the answers to all such questions of moral necessity require the anthropologist to use his or her own conscience in view of the facts observed and the likely consequences of the action taken. One must weigh the various courses of action, and choose what appeals most to one's own conscience. In this weighing process, several likelihoods need to be considered, such as:

- *Resistance to change:* Getting people to change long-standing behaviors is usually extremely difficult. The effort to *correct* practices might consume a great deal of time, resources, and good will, only to produce nothing in the long run. (Out of respect for the researcher, people often agree outwardly to his or her demands, only to continue their customs in private.)

- *Interrelatedness of customs:* Nearly all customary behavior is an integral part of a far-reaching, coherent system of custom and belief that helps to satisfy important needs. Changing one element of this system is very likely to produce unexpected and unwanted results. For example, the practice of female genital mutilation is an important expression of the authority of older people, especially women, in some Middle Eastern cultures. Simply stopping the practice could have the effect of shifting authority to health workers and younger women, thereby seriously weakening the whole structure of the traditional culture. In opposing the practice, one must consider whether the outcome is worth this risk.

- *The loss of identities:* In today's world, the traditions and customs of many local communities are being lost, as world commerce and communication expands, and as national and international interests seek increased control over peoples and their environments. Young people in many places are more exposed to the culture and technology of the dominant industrial world than they are to their own local traditions. This has many troubling results, among them a loss of ethnic pride, a new perception of their own past as worthless, and a sense of confusion and purposelessness about the future. Many traditional communities are fighting back against this trend, trying to revive their customs and their pride. Any attempt to question local customs must take these facts into account.

TAKING ROLES, FITTING IN

We have looked at the basic ethical standards that apply to all anthropological field work. Now we are ready to discuss further details of how to manage relationships in the field. Usually the people that we study are not familiar at first with what we anthropologists do or how we think. They are curious about us, and they also are likely to feel unsure of how much to trust us, and how to conduct themselves in our presence. They want to know the same kinds of things about us that we want to know about the people we associate with or do business with. What do we want from them? What do we think about them? What are our values? Who are our friends? What kind of help, support, advice, or friendship can we offer them? How long will we be here? What will be the consequences for them of our work?

In order to build trusting relationships with people and to minimize the awkwardness that people usually feel dealing with strangers, it is important that the researcher's behavior should make sense within the range of people's expectations, reflect locally accepted values in the sense that one is seen as a "decent person," or "someone we would not mind having around," and be consistent and at least somewhat predictable. In other words, the researcher should try to learn as quickly as possible what the recognizable, respectable roles are in this community that fit with the work he or she needs to do.

This might turn out to be quite simple, or it might not. If the researcher, or the agency for whom he works, has a history of friendly relations with the community, it might only be necessary to explain to residents what a new research project is about, and how one plans to do it, and ask for their comments and suggestions. At the other extreme, if there are serious rivalries within the community, or a history of unhappy relationships with outsiders, or mistrust of the sponsoring organization, or if the topic of the research is the subject of strong emotions, the process of selecting a role might be complex and difficult. First, let us examine some of the advantages and disadvantages of various kinds of roles, then turn to the topic of how to deal with especially difficult research situations.

CLOTHING, SPEECH, MANNERS

For purposes of research, it is best to dress, speak, and conduct oneself as much as possible like an ordinary member of the study community. Clothes that signify a social class, ethnic background, profession, religion, or life-style that is different than those of the average community member only serve to increase the social distance between researcher and community, and should be avoided. This is true even if, or especially if, the researcher usually wears an official uniform in her work. Usually, people feel honored and at ease when the researcher makes an effort to adhere to their customs. If for some reason the local dress cannot be worn, it is at least important to wear clothes that are not considered indecent, inappropriate, or silly. Even though shorts and sandals are more comfortable in tropical Latin America, when doing field work I wear long pants and shoes like virtually all the men my age.

Likewise, it is extremely difficult to conduct good anthropological research unless one speaks the local language reasonably well. If the researcher speaks a different dialect of the same language, it is helpful to learn and use the local variations, if not of pronunciation, at least of vocabulary. (But be careful – some local words have dangerous double meanings, and some that you may hear frequently are nevertheless considered rude!)

Of course, the same goes for manners. One should do one's best from the beginning to learn the rules about when to stand or sit, how to greet people and say goodbye, how to express thanks or give respect, what kind of gifts to give and when, and what behaviors annoy or shock people. One must avoid showing shock or displeasure when local customs violate one's own norms, as well. To the extent you can, eat what the community eats, rise and sleep when they do, learn their games and pastimes.

EXAMPLES OF ROLES

Within these general rules, there are a number of possible ways to present oneself to the study community. What are the distinct roles recognized by members of the community? Government official? Laborer? Healer? Entertainer? Priest? Teacher? Housewife? Storekeeper? Farmer? Which roles make the most sense to local people, given the kind of work the researcher does?

The Role of Student or Scholar

Often the best role an anthropological researcher can take in a community is that of student or scholar. Except for those who live in remote rural settings, most people are familiar with this role. They know at least in general what it means to collect information for a scientific study. They have an image of a scholar as someone well trained in collecting information, and usually more or less trustworthy. The advantages of this role, then, are the following:

1. This is usually the most honest way to present oneself. The researcher, after all, is a student of the local culture and community, and usually is a professional scholar in some sense of the word as well.
2. Scholars tend to be understood, respected, and trusted (although there are exceptions).
3. Part of a scholar's job is to observe and learn. It usually makes sense to people that such a person wants to take part in everything, observe everything, and ask questions. People will often set

aside local customs that would prohibit a relative stranger from participating or asking, because they understand this.

4. As an outsider with no reason to take sides in community conflicts or to align herself with a clique, some people might trust a scholar with information they would not give to their neighbors.

5. The outsider status of the scholar also helps people keep a certain emotional distance with respect to the researcher. This can help to avoid conflicts and disappointments that might develop if the researcher is seen in a more intimate role. Note that this is different from the exaggerated *emotional objectivity* of positivist science, in which the researcher seeks to suppress all feelings about the research topic.

6. Especially, it is natural for the scholar to show humility, patience, and deference in dealing with the research community, qualities that build rapport better than any others I know. It is human nature to enjoy teaching someone who wants to learn one's ideas, knowledge and skills.

The disadvantages of the scholar role also result from one's reputation as being a fairly high status, neutral outsider, and include the following:

1. Some people may be sensitive to the scholar's high status and education, and might conceal things about their lives that they consider humiliating, especially things they believe mark them as poor or uneducated. They might behave more formally in the researcher's presence than at other times as well.

2. Similarly, the scholar role creates some danger that the researcher will be identified with high status members of the research locale. This can be serious, because there are usually long standing barriers to communication between high and low status people in a community. A researcher who is firmly identified with the higher status group will have trouble accessing facts or observing settings that are protected by this barrier. These two problems are precisely why humility is so important in the researcher role.

3. In some cultures, it is customary to honor scholars with gifts and ceremonies. This can create a moral hazard, when people with barely enough resources feel they must share what they have generously with the researcher. It might be necessary to explain carefully that one honors these customs but according to one's professional culture, one cannot receive gifts without paying for them.

The Role of Friend

In the course of doing anthropological field work, it is very natural to develop close relationships with some members of the study community, especially with *key informants* (see Chapter Seven). Friendship is a universal human bond that often grows between people who live and work closely together. We learn to recognize and appreciate each other's ideas, needs, skills, and feelings. We learn to feel grateful for each other's recognition and support. *In situations where this is natural, I believe it is a mistake to try to avoid it.* However, friendship can be a serious hazard to anthropological research under certain circumstances, and one needs to take these into account.

The advantages of the role of friend are pretty obvious. A friend is a deeply trusted person with whom we can discuss a wide range of subjects comfortably, a person to whom we can show sides of our lives and personalities we would not show to many others. Besides, a friend is generally someone whose company we enjoy. It is not a burden to set aside time to be with such a person, even when we are busy. The learning value of this relationship can be enormous. There are two major disadvantages of the friendship role.

First, friendship implies mutual obligation, sometimes very heavy obligation. If I behave as someone's friend, I invite that person to rely on me for help. The extent and kind of help will depend on the culture, but friends in many cultures might expect you to loan or give them money, share your personal resources (car, bike, or horse, computer, tools, food, telephone, garden products, etc.), join with them in their disputes, spend your leisure time with them, share their work, or make yourself available to them at any hour of the day or night. Failure to honor such customs might mean the end of the friendship.

Second, consider the maxim, "the friend of my enemy is my enemy." When there are serious conflicts or communication barriers within a community, taking the role of friend with one person or group might mean losing the trust of another.

For example, I know an anthropologist who wanted to study land inheritance in a rural Scottish village. She observed the way neighbors and friends behaved toward each other – inviting one another to dinner, bringing gifts, and so on – and she began to take this role with one family after another in the village. After several months, she discovered that most of the people she interviewed were giving her false information about how much land they had, and how they had gotten it. It turned out that there was a custom in this part of Scotland that one does not reveal these things to one's neighbors. Because each family soon saw her as the friend of the family down the road, she could not get the data she needed for her study, and eventually had to abandon it.

In general, then, the researcher should let friendships evolve slowly and naturally, and avoid choosing close friends before knowing what the various factions and alliances are in the community, and something about the rules governing friendship. It is possible to be friendly and helpful in a general way, without choosing favorites or committing oneself to deep mutual obligations.

The role of *lover* can be considered a special category of friend, which may have some of the same advantages, but also has some big additional disadvantages. Need I say more?

The Roles of Leader, Teacher, and Expert

The anthropologist is likely to have more formal education than the average person in the study community, and higher social status. Depending on the researcher's age, sex, and title, the status difference can be minor, or it can be quite dramatic. In either case, it is not at all unusual for some people in the study community to look to the researcher for leadership and help, at least occasionally. When this happens, it can be very difficult to avoid taking on the role of leader, teacher, or expert advisor. For one thing, the anthropologist does not want to disappoint the people she is working with. For another thing, it feels good to be admired and appreciated.

For health workers, especially in a traditional society where such people are highly respected, it is a double temptation to take on leadership roles. One is trained to exercise such roles, and it becomes part of one's normal behavior when working with non-experts in the field of health. The titles, uniforms, equipment, work environment, and pay of a health worker often place him or her automatically in a position of leadership in the eyes of many people.

In Chapter Eleven, we will discuss the special case of action anthropology, where the researcher might seek to combine the roles of participant observer and leader. For ordinary ethnographic work, by now it should be no surprise that I warn against taking on these roles if possible. I also suggest keeping a low profile if one must assume such roles. The best strategy is to help others recognize their own knowledge and talents, and arrange for them to take the credit for leading and problem solving. If one is a stranger in the community, it might not be difficult to do this, but if one is already known, for example as a health worker or teacher, it might require a long period of *transferring leadership to others* for the researcher to develop an effective role.

The advantages of the leader/teacher role are twofold. First, if one is successful at solving problems one earns the gratitude and admiration of at least some people in the community (possibly alienating others, however). Second, the strong status of a recognized leader may give the researcher access to people, settings, and information that he/she would not otherwise get (and possibly lose access to other sources, however).

There are, however, numerous disadvantages associated with this role. To the extent that the researcher accepts a leadership role, people's expectations of him or her will grow. If one is not successful (often a bigger possibility than we imagine), one stands to lose respect, status, and good will in the community. If there are factions or disagreements in the community (and there almost always are), a leader will be pressured to take sides. Each faction will seek to recruit to its own cause the prestige and power that goes with leadership. Obviously, taking sides can destroy the researcher's effectiveness as a scientist, by closing off access to important information and contacts.

I have emphasized the importance of humility and the role of the learner for effective naturalistic research. Although it is possible to lead and still be humble, it is far more difficult for others to perceive leaders as equals and as learners. People have a tendency to show respect to leaders, to try to make an impression on them, and to assume that they know things that they may in fact need to know.

Competitiveness is a very common human trait. In almost any community, there are those who enjoy their ability to influence others, and those who dream of being leaders themselves. Most such people find it easy to criticize and obstruct others who share influence.

As practical advice on how to handle the status of well-educated outsider, then:

1. *Avoid association with symbols of status and power*, such as wearing a uniform, carrying technical equipment, using expensive transportation, housing, food, jewelry, or clothes, using technical language or concepts, and having the demeanor and speech habits of a teacher or leader.
2. *Avoid close association with powerful people*, such as political figures, religious elites, high-level bureaucrats, local celebrities, or very wealthy residents.
3. *Make opportunities to give leadership and credit to others*, especially when people are inclined to give these things to you. Be

especially sensitive to those who already have some stature as leaders in the community.

4. *Don't be afraid to show your ignorance or ask for help*, thereby supporting others' self esteem.

CULTURE SHOCK: UNAVOIDABLE, HIGHLY VALUABLE

I was teaching a course at a nursing college in Thailand, and when the course was over, the students and other faculty arranged for a big celebration, with food, drink, and music. I expected to sit quietly at my table and enjoy the performance. Early in the evening, it became clear that the class had a very different plan. I must get up and sing. They had hired an orchestra that knew how to play hundreds of Western tunes, so I would have plenty of chance to show off my talents. At the age of sixty-five, I had never gotten up and sung in front of a ballroom full of people in my whole life, and I was completely petrified. But there was no way to get out of it. Moreover, I did not know any of the tunes the band knew, and ended up having to sing *Amazing Grace* a capella, the sweat running down my face and my voice trembling.

What I had experienced was a mild form of culture shock. Thais in leadership positions are accustomed to taking an active role in whatever festivities are underway. Not to do so is unthinkable to them. From this I learned two important things: First, next time I go to Thailand I will make sure I have practiced a variety of popular tunes. Second, the concepts of respect and status are very different in Thailand and the United States. Here, we accord people status based on how well they can perform the specific art or profession they were trained for. In Thailand, a high-status person is respected for his or her position itself, not just for whatever abilities he might have. This means taking a leadership position in all kinds of activities, regardless of one's training or specialty. Knowing this, high-status Thais of course make a point of mastering the skills needed in such situations.

No discussion about the role of the observer in a strange community would be complete without attention to *culture shock*. This refers to a range of feelings that arise when we become actively involved in events that are unexpected and confusing. It happens to every anthropologist, often many times during the course of a career. It is often very unpleasant, but it is usually extremely valuable also, because it involves rapid learning. In doing anthropological research, one must expect to experience culture shock from time to time. There is really no way to avoid it. The important points here are two:

First, be aware that you will make cultural mistakes or fail to anticipate situations, simply because you are not familiar with the assumptions
and rules of the culture you are studying.

Second, when you do experience culture shock, look for the valuable
lesson that the incident contains. Ask yourself *why* you were embarrassed,
or failed to anticipate what happened – how your assumptions differed
from those of the people around you, and why.

IF YOUR TIME IN THE COMMUNITY IS LIMITED

Some researchers are not able to arrange ideal conditions for doing naturalistic anthropological studies. Their job and family might be located
in a community far from the one they are studying, or they might be required to study several communities at the same time, or they might have
only a few months in which to prepare, carry out, and analyze a research
project. In some cases, the research director scarcely spends any time in
the study community, taking the role of directing one or more assistants
to actually do the research.

In these cases, the researcher's objective should be to seek ways of
duplicating as closely as possible the ideal roles presented here. Here are
some general ideas that might help guide a nonresident researcher in this
effort:

1. *Find ways to get to know the community before beginning data
   collection.* Whatever the reason that the researcher cannot live in
   the community, there are things that he or she can do to become
   familiar with it. Visits to the community to observe its physical
   setting, interviews with a wide variety of residents, library research
   on the history of the area and the people, and the study of public
   records on population, health, economics, environment, land use,
   and so on, are all very helpful.
2. *Use as many sources of information as you can.* If you observe or
   talk to people who live or work in the community, do not limit
   yourself only to leaders (teachers, politicians or leaders, officials or
   health workers, priests, wealthy landlords). Talk to older people,
   younger people, and children. Talk to people in different occupations and different ethnic groups. If there are migrant workers in
   the community, talk to them. Check what people tell you against
   other sources of data, such as government or clinic records. If
   there are several organizations in the community, try to get each
   of their perspectives as well.

3. *Train assistants in advance in the principles of participant observation outlined here.* Whether you are using hired assistants or students, never send them to the study community until they have been carefully trained in these principles. Simply reading the principles may not be enough. Observation and practice might also be necessary.

4. *Make good use of key informants.* The concept of *key informant* is discussed in the next chapter. A non-resident researcher can often form a close relationship with one or more key informants in the community and keep close contact with them. This can be extremely valuable to identify and correct problems with the research early. In some cases it might be wise to recruit and pay one or more residents, who can act as key informants. However, such people must be chosen very carefully (see Chapter Seven).

5. *Collect and analyze data at the same time.* The power of the naturalistic method is that every new bit of information clarifies the research problem and leads to more intelligent questions. The non-resident researcher, like the true participant observer, needs to be constantly adjusting the data collection to fit her evolving intuition of the problem.

6. *Pay close attention to your own and your assistants' reputation and acceptance in the community.* Find ways to build your reputation and those of your assistants that do not take a great deal of work time. Volunteer work with the community, participation in social events, spending leisure time with people, attending church or temple, or shopping in the community, all are helpful.

7. *Be careful not to use status or authority to coerce cooperation.* As an educator or health provider, you will be tempted to take short cuts to secure people's cooperation, by simply using your status or authority. This is one of the most serious mistakes researchers can make. If people cooperate without genuine trust and acceptance, the information they provide will be of questionable value. Their level of cooperation may dramatically decline over time, as they begin to feel more and more exploited. They might be susceptible to pressure from elements in the community to withdraw their cooperation, or even to actively sabotage the project.

8. *Keep your relationship with the community fresh after the research.* Once you have done the work of building rapport and gathering data, you will be in a position to work in the same community much more efficiently in the future. By keeping your relationships active, you will also learn new things that bear on your original research, and you can continue to refine it. One

excellent way to do this is to donate your services to the community (if they want you to!) as a consultant on issues you feel you understand.

I am well aware that all of these measures require careful preparation, thought, sustained effort, and above all *time*. Unfortunately, I do not believe there is any way to do good anthropology quickly.

THE RESEARCHER BEYOND THE COMMUNITY

A scholar is, almost by definition, a member of a community of scholars. Whatever one's discipline – physics, literature, music, biology, nursing, or anthropology – one's work is most appreciated by those who have mastered the same techniques and read the same books as oneself. Even the solitary researcher uses the journals and conferences of her discipline to engage others interested in similar issues. Success in one's profession depends on the approval of one's fellow professionals.

This does not mean that social scientists are unconcerned about the impact of their work on the communities they study. Many books have been written about our moral duties in this respect. However, because of the strong dependencies that link scholars, we social scientists have always been inclined to put high importance on the scholarly uses of our research. Whatever other values we have, we aim to produce lectures and publishable reports that will interest our colleagues and advance our careers. We strive to produce material useful in our classrooms. But, because our work often has the power to influence what actually happens in our study communities, we are at risk of committing unconscious moral mistakes.

It is human nature to believe that our lives are beneficial to society, that our personal goals at least do no harm to others, and usually actually help people. Most of us have the habit of seeing the beneficial side of what we do, and remain unconscious of its possible cost to others.

For example, the biological researcher delights in producing a useful new drug, feeling that his work is an unmixed blessing for human kind. He might be insulted if you pointed out to him that his invention is only useful for a rare disease, that it is very expensive and will probably not be available to poor people, and that the money used to develop it might have been used to save thousands of lives by providing very simple things like clean water and food to those who lack them. Indeed, who would be rude enough to say such things?

Similarly, the social scientist feels the same pride in her skill and hard work, showing her colleagues how high school test scores are more closely related to the children's home environment than to the conditions in the schools themselves. She hopes this will lead to better education for parents, so they can help their children at home. Instead, it ends up helping those who argue against better funding for public schools.

I believe it is too much to ask that anthropologists place a higher value on their study communities than on their colleagues as audiences for their work. If we demanded this, we might discourage able people from doing anthropology at all. However, for several reasons I do think the researcher should try to balance the benefits of her work to these two audiences. First, I believe that joining a community in order to study it actually does amount to a commitment to contribute what one can to that community. This is simple everyday ethics. Second, the researcher, by virtue of her education, status, and connections to outside agencies and scholars, may have knowledge and power that members of the community lack. The failure to use these resources when able to do so is, in my view, a sign of selfishness. This in turn requires the researcher to think about this issue, to study the possibilities outside the community for using her knowledge in a beneficial way. Third, in the long run, putting a high priority on the possible benefits to the community builds trust between researchers and communities. This can help the individual researcher in future dealings with the same community, and it can ultimately help other researchers in this and other communities.

Some ideas about how to fulfill this obligation to one's research community include the following:

1. Share the results of your research with members of the community. Invite them to comment on it, and to use it in their own work. (Here, one must be careful not to give unfair advantage to one faction or interest group over another. If there is a chance that one's findings might be abused by members of the group, this step might not be possible.)
2. When you write reports of your research, imagine who might use the information, and for what purposes. If you don't like the possible consequences for the community, figure out how to minimize them. Note that this step is in keeping with the naturalistic theory of knowledge, even though positivist social scientists might disagree with it. Imagine also that members of the community themselves are receiving these reports. How will they react? Again, if their reaction will be negative (and you cannot always guess accurately), you must decide whether the positive uses of the findings for them will outweigh the negative.
3. Think about specific ways in which your community is exploited by outside groups. How can you use your knowledge to counteract this exploitation?

4. Join (or start!) organizations working to promote the well-being of your community and those like it. Lend your knowledge and skill to these efforts.

SUMMARY

We will return to consider the role of the researcher in and beyond the community in Chapter Eleven, Action Anthropology. The main points of this chapter are that:

- the naturalistic researcher's goal is to understand behavior in its natural settings and interrelationships;
- as such, his or her goal is to participate in and observe those settings and relationships with as little distorting effect as possible;
- the natural way to do this is to learn as quickly as possible what behaviors are understandable and acceptable in the community, and adapt these as best one can to the data collection tasks;
- behaving as a member of the community means participating in relationships based on normal expectations and feelings, and it obligates the researcher to take those expectations and feelings seriously and do one's best to honor them, especially when the social status and resources of the researcher are distinctly greater than those of the average community member; and
- although far from the distant objectivity of the positivist ideal, these instructions fit well with the naturalistic theory of knowledge.

CHAPTER SEVEN

Collecting Data

GUIDE TO THIS CHAPTER

This chapter is meant to help new researchers understand how to collect and analyze anthropological material, offering some ideas and suggestions my students and I have found useful over the years.

There are already many books on how to collect and analyze anthropological material. Most of these are full of good suggestions that fit well with the naturalistic way of working. Also, every anthropological field worker has a unique personality, set of skills, and favorite way of working. There is no *one best way* to do these tasks. Each researcher needs to discover through practice what works best for him or her.

In Chapter Five, we discussed research design, and the importance of selecting a good research problem. Here, we talk more about the process of identifying and filling in the needed knowledge in order to answer the problem question.

It is important to remember that our sense of the problem grows and changes as the data collection process goes forward. We do not try to force our observations to conform to the original intuition. Rather, we keep asking whether our intuition seems to be supported by the data, and changing it when the data show convincingly that our original understanding will not lead us to the most useful answers. We do not wait until the data collection is *finished* to raise questions about our problem, our approach, our intuition, or our design.

Parts of the data collection process include:

- background research on the historical, geographic, economic, and political context of the study, which helps us understand the meaning of many observations, how they are related to one another, and what kinds of action might be needed to change them;
- a study of the physical community and population – terrain, buildings, resources, and the main characteristics of the people, such as

age, gender, race and culture, occupation, and physical and mental health;

- an investigation of the social organization and people's roles in the community, which help us to determine the lines of authority, friendship, cooperation, competition, and conflict; who has a personal interest in the issues that we are studying, and what that interest is.

This chapter also contains advice on how to choose situations to observe, how to choose interviewees, what to ask, and how to do an open-ended interview. Suggestions about how to record data are also included.

We discuss the important fact that an interview does not represent *facts* or opinions or beliefs that were already there in the mind of the interviewee. Rather, an interview is a creative process, in which each participant is creating a narrative that makes sense at that time, in that place, and with those people. It is the job of the researcher to understand, using all the available data, why someone constructed that particular narrative, not what fixed *truth* is contained in the narrative itself.

PLANNING FOR RESEARCH

Before undertaking an anthropological project, you must propose a research problem and conduct background research.

The Research Problem

Of course the most important step in planning for anthropological research is to select and develop the research problem. In Chapters Three, Four, and Five, we showed that the problem selection process is more complex and difficult than most researchers (and research teachers) realize. Many projects fail because the problem was not well formed and the methods were not well suited to achieving an answer.

Without repeating that discussion here, it is worth noting that *one's knowledge about the research community and one's sense of the research problem generally develop together*, they are part of an ongoing process that is never completely finished. Choosing a problem is not a single grand decision, like buying a house; it is a process of developing and refining an intuition.

Occasionally the anthropologist must begin field work with very little background knowledge, having been assigned a place to study and a problem. In that case, background research and on-site data collection must begin simultaneously. Usually this is not the case, though, and it is best to learn a good deal about one's research community before beginning a focused research project. This idea is not so strange when we consider that a chemist or biologist also learns a great deal about the specific topic he or she will research even before applying for funds to study it. Note, however, that naturalistic research seeks to understand communities as unique patterns, and it is not enough to know something about human communities, or even about the national culture, social class, occupations, or ethnicity of the people one is going to study. A corollary of this principle is that anthropological research takes a long time to do adequately.

Background Research

One can learn many useful things about a research community before beginning intensive field work. Visits to the site, conversations with people who live or have lived there, interviews with public officials who serve the area, and study of public records are all useful. The types of data one is able to assemble vary from place to place, of course. General topics for background research include the following:

The History of the Area and the Culture

Communities do not appear in their present form out of nowhere. Every group and every locale has a history that must be understood if one is to understand the present dynamics of life. The way people behave grows from, to a great extent, their understanding of who they are, what their community is, and how things got that way. Why are certain families looked up to, even though they might be poor? Why do relationships between one group and another appear incurably hostile, for no apparent reason? What determines which local habits are terribly important to people and which get little notice? What are the dominant occupations in this area, and why? What have been the major social changes in the past few years, and how has that affected people's lives?

EXAMPLE: Adjoining Neighborhoods: Different Histories, Different Problems

In a community where I once did research, there are two low-income neighborhoods side by side, separated by a busy street I will call Hill Street. They are about the same size, and both have been there for many years. In the neighborhood east of Hill Street, there are strong organizations on most blocks that bind neighbors together in cooperative projects and political unity. There is relatively little crime in this area, and the streets are well kept and attractive. Residents and visitors alike generally speak well of the immediate area.

By contrast, the neighborhood on the west side of Hill Street has fewer and weaker organizations, and as a result there are more social problems. The City has approved the building of many small rental apartments on the west side, and the residents of these units often do not stay long. There is a serious problem here with drug use and crime.

What accounts for this puzzling difference? A little research on their history reveals that the east side was settled about a century ago mainly by members of a single strong labor union. These were people who had steady incomes, were proud of their work, and felt strong ties to each other. For many years they fought off attempts by the City to locate apartment buildings there. They kept close watch on the streets and demanded effective policing when trouble appeared. Residents felt public pressure to keep their homes looking nice.

The west side of Hill Street developed a few years later, around a train stop where residents could board to get to their jobs in nearby cities. The people were similar in income, but had different and less stable jobs. From the early days, there was more movement in and out of the west side neighborhood, and fewer close ties among neighbors.

Nowadays, hardly anyone remembers these historical details. The labor union of the east side is long gone, and people on both sides of Hill Street have the same sorts of jobs. But the attitude of pride and solidarity that has been part of the east neighborhood's tradition still remains. It has been built into the physical and moral landscape in forms such as housing, parks, trees, and well-kept streets, as well as alert, proud, and cooperative residents. A forgotten history, once known, greatly clarifies the difference between the east and the west sides.

The Physical Community and Population

Much can be learned about a community by studying its physical attributes and population. Maps should be made or found to locate physical features such as housing, water, roads, public buildings, businesses, schools, churches and temples, playgrounds and parks, forests, fields and crops, transport routes, medical facilities and other features of possible interest. If one is doing a health study, it might be possible to map illnesses, sanitation problems, and other health hazards. In many places, local government offices list population by age and gender, household composition, occupation, land ownership, and other features. Police often keep records of crimes and accidents by area.

Casual observation can provide information about the condition of buildings, differences between neighborhoods, the apparent age and wealth or poverty of the people, ethnic differences (food, clothing, language), local occupations, local animals, popular products and stores, modes of transport, and outdoor pastimes. Signs of social stress, such as vandalism, bars on windows and locks on doors, graffiti, drunkenness, street idleness, trash, abandoned buildings, and vacant lots – or the absence of these things – are instructive.

Social Organization

By the social organization of a community, we mean the systematic ways that people relate to one another, and the categories and ideas they use as guidelines for interaction. The broad categories of social organization are kinship, residence patterns, social status, age and gender distinctions, voluntary associations, social networks, cliques and factions, ethnic and religious groups, social class relations, and leadership.

These together make up a very large and complex set of relationships and rules in most communities, and it usually takes many months to do a thorough study. However, it is useful to know some general features of social organization before beginning formal research. Some extremely useful background questions are as follows:

1. What is the actual (not just the formal) leadership structure of the area? Who makes collective decisions, and about what? Who are the opinion leaders, and what do they believe? Whose approval is needed for what actions? Who controls what resources?
2. What is the composition of families and households?
3. What are the more important voluntary associations and cooperative networks, what people are involved in them, what are their roles in the community, and what are some of their concerns and beliefs?
4. What ethnic and religious divisions are there in the community? What are the relationships between them like?

Armed with answers to questions such as these, the researcher can begin to plan where to look for various kinds of information, who to approach (and who to avoid) about helping to get the project accepted in the community, and even what some of the community's health problems are likely to be.

OBSERVING AND TAKING NOTES

As the phrase *participant observation* implies, most of anthropological field work consists of taking part in community life, while observing it systematically. Of course, "observation" often entails listening and questioning, and sometimes also recording on film, audiotape, or videotape. Occasionally, the observer will even take measurements or samples of materials for later analysis.

In Chapter Eleven, we will discuss a style of working, *action anthropology*, in which one of the goals is to actually contribute to changing the community. Here, we will discuss ordinary data collection through observation, which has four main goals:

- to record a representative variety of cultural behaviors, contexts, and meanings relevant to the research problem;
- to minimize the distortion of normal behavior caused by observing;
- to record accurately what one sees and hears; and,
- to maintain rapport between the observer and the community.

General Principles of Observation

In Chapter Six we talked about the roles anthropologists can take in order to make the process of observation as easy and as accurate as possible. Of course, public life is relatively easy to observe in most communities, especially if one plays a helping role. However, the more private a behavior or setting is, the more these four goals are likely to conflict with each other. The desire to observe intimate settings makes rapport more difficult and distortion more likely. Accurate recording on-the-spot might make participants feel self-conscious, again affecting both naturalness and rapport. One must balance each goal against the others, and there is no formula for doing this. One must usually rely on one's social skills, experience, and judgment. A few general rules might help, however:

1. Choose your level and style of participation carefully. Use your social skills to "read" each situation and decide how much to participate. In many situations, staying quietly in the background is best. However, taking part in public recreation or group work, such as some team sports, dancing, agricultural or construction projects, for example, are typical *hands-on* observation situations, where not taking part might send the wrong signal. The same goes for asking questions. Your basic social experience should help you know when questions are acceptable, and what kind of questions.
2. Expect culture shock and embarrassment. As a relative newcomer to the community, you cannot be expected to know what is appropriate all the time, and you will make embarrassing mistakes. Arriving at a gathering at the wrong time, or dressed wrong, or lacking the right supplies or gifts are common, as is saying the wrong thing to the wrong person, using the wrong gestures or posture, laughing at serious situations and failing to laugh at funny ones – all this is part of culture shock (see Chapter Six).
3. Take ample time to establish rapport and trust, even before openly observing public settings, and especially before intruding on more

private ones. Overlooking this need is a very common mistake in planning ethnographic research. In Chapters Two through Six, we emphasized the critical roles of emotion and meaning in the understanding of culture. To arrive at a process through which these features of the community can be seen and understood, the researcher must normalize his or her role as much as possible, and this generally takes weeks to months of background work.

4. Minimize openly recording data unless it is a normal part of the activity (for example, health care, advising, or teaching) in which you are engaged. Take notes in private where possible. If you have permission to use audio or video recording, try to do so delicately. Never do so without permission from all participants.

What Situations and Behaviors to Observe

In Chapter Five we discussed the problem of what questions to ask, and to a large extent, your questions will suggest what situations you should make an effort to see. One good way of stating this is to ask, "What contrasts do I want to understand?"

If you are interested in the elderly, for example, it may be less important for you to spend time watching school activities or children's games, but not necessarily. Suppose you find out that elderly grandparents are very concerned about what the children do, or do not do, in school. Then you might actually want to look for the source of their concern, in order to find out whether it is realistic or not, what it is that worries them about it, or what, if anything, might be done about it.

Also, there is the very important matter of understanding broad cultural patterns that are revealed by observing many seemingly unrelated situations.

EXAMPLE: U.S. and Japan:
Diverse Cultural Attitudes Toward Passivity

Japan and the United States have very different attitudes toward passive relaxation. This difference is very important to understanding health behavior in the two cultures, but one must observe many different kinds of situations in order to realize its strength.

- *Americans typically experience being sick, even a little, as an anxiety producing situation in which they cannot do the normal physical activities of everyday life. Being "idle" or "weak" are highly feared self-perceptions. Japanese, in contrast, tend to take small illnesses in stride, actively enjoying the opportunity to be passively taken care of.*

- *Americans tend to become bored and irritable if they have to sit in one place for several hours. On American passenger planes, the flight crew must work hard, serving drinks and food, showing movies, joking with the bored passengers to keep them happy. In Japan, most airplane and train passengers on long trips simply go to sleep, showing their comfort with the passive position they find themselves in.*
- *American parents are most pleased when their young babies are more active, alert, playful, and talkative than other children. They spend a lot of time trying to make the children laugh, play, and make sounds. Japanese parents admire quiet, passive babies, and spend equal amounts of time soothing and quieting their children.*
- *Most American art forms strive to excite the audience's emotions. A good piece of art, architecture, literature, or performance is often said to be "dynamic," or "exciting." Many (not all) Japanese art forms take the opposite approach, seeking to produce feelings of peaceful harmony and balance.*

Accordingly, a good field anthropologist tries to observe and record as widely as possible. It might be said that looking for cultural information in every situation becomes a habit that one practices continually. Gradually the anthropologist develops a *way of seeing* that is automatically attuned to the patterns of life. Whenever I find myself in a new place, I now have a habit observing what is unusual, and playing with explanations of why. This is what we might call the *anthropological eye*.

EXAMPLE: *Havana Street Scene Suggests Social Stability*

Because of the U.S.-led embargo against trade, in the year 2002 Cuba was a society very different from most of those I was familiar with. Just walking down a busy street in Havana with my anthropological eyes open, I could notice things with profound meaning. For example, most of the shops had no signs of any kind – no advertising, not even a shop name on the door. Yet shoppers came and went just as in any big city. It struck me that everyone who shopped here knew from experience what goods were sold in which stores. This in turn led me to hypothesize several other things:

1. *The relationships between the sellers and the buyers must be, on the average, more intimate than they are in more commercialized places. This might promote fairness in trade practices.*
2. *The variety and quantity of goods for sale must be far smaller than in other cities. This fits with the commercial isolation of Havana.*
3. *The cost of advertising and marketing these goods must be far lower here – a larger proportion of the cost must be going to the maker and the merchant.*
4. *Most of the people who shop here must live fairly nearby, in order to know this street so well. The cost of transport must be much less than*

in comparable large cities elsewhere. I did in fact notice that there were hardly any places for people to park a car in the area.

5. *If everyone is so familiar with this neighborhood, the likelihood of meeting someone you know must be much greater than in other places. In fact, I did notice that people tended to greet each other in the street a good deal. People were even quick to make eye contact with me, a complete stranger.*

6. *This familiarity must have the effect of greatly reducing crime. In fact, Havana has almost no violent crime in spite of severe poverty.*

Many other such details came to my attention as well: Shop windows often contain a television set tuned to a sports event. This usually draws a crowd (sometimes a very large and noisy one), implying: (a) that many Cubans do not have their own televisions; (b) that many Cubans love sports; and, (c) that Cubans trust each other enough to feel comfortable in a crowd of relative strangers. This was confirmed (in part) by seeing pretty young women hitchhiking in downtown Havana – something one never sees in the United States.

Try to observe situations that contrast important dimensions of your intuition. In Chapter Five we discussed the importance of asking questions that focus on theoretically rich contrasts. We used the example of *sexual pressure as a source of stress among young women*, suggesting that one would want to vary stress levels, gender, and age, in order to understand this problem better. If you study alcohol use, try to observe situations where people drink and similar ones where they do not. Try to learn about the family lives, recreation, and work of people who drink a lot and those of a similar age, gender, and occupation who do not.

Minimizing Distortion

Obviously, the less the interviewer's presence interferes with the natural situation, the less distorted it will be. One must use one's experience and social skills to judge the impact one is having on a situation, and adjust one's behavior accordingly. In public settings, taking part in the normal activity is often less disruptive than silently watching, but not always. In more private settings, one must usually do two things: first, spend time establishing trust with the participants before trying to observe; and second, fit in to the setting quietly. Some times it is possible to observe without being seen or noticed at all, but this is of course risky, as people might be offended if they find out.

In any case, one must balance the goal of neutrality with the goals of thoroughness, rapport, and accurate recording. It is sometimes more important to be a slightly disruptive observer or participant, than not to observe at all. A clumsy performance of a group activity by the researcher might disrupt the activity thoroughly, but might win the observer a large measure of acceptance in the community that will more than compensate for the disruption. One must use one's judgment.

Rapport Building

We have already discussed rapport building at some length in Chapter Six. Here we only need to say that one must spend significant time in the community building rapport before trying to observe sensitive situations. By the same token, obtrusive observing by a mistrusted researcher can damage rapport so severely that one might be later excluded even from mundane activities.

KEEPING RECORDS

Good ethnographers develop their own ways of keeping records, ways that balance accuracy, efficiency, and convenience for them. Here are some suggestions that my students and I have found useful.

Audio and Video Recordings

Audio and video recordings provide the most accurate records, but have two serious disadvantages. First, they are usually somewhat intrusive and might both introduce distortion into behavior and injure rapport. Second, being linear in time, they are extremely time-consuming to analyze. Digital coding might help, but I find that having written notes that I can scan with my own eyes is a far more efficient medium.

Audiotapes can be transcribed into print, but transcription is extremely time consuming (figure at least two hours of transcribing for every hour of tape). Tapes are most useful as (a) backup materials to clarify one's written notes; (b) a means to record extremely complex and fast-moving activities where note taking simply cannot capture the important details; and/or (c) a way to record events where the taping process is scarcely noticeable, as for example at public ceremonies.

Taking Notes

I find that being able to take abbreviated or shorthand notes rapidly is the most efficient way to record most kinds of observations, provided I always go over my notes the same day and fill in details while they are still fresh in my memory. This requirement, together with that of adding comments (as discussed in more detail later), makes it especially useful to leave ample space in the notebook for the addition of details and comments.

One of the important principles of good note taking is the careful inclusion of context. At the very least, every notebook entry should note:

- the date, day of the week, and time of day of the event;
- the location of the event;
- the names of those present; and,
- the purpose of the activity observed.

To this list it is often useful to add further context, such as the weather, mood of participants, and preceding events that led to the activity. There are two reasons for including such contextual information. First, it helps directly with the analysis of similarities and differences among the variables of time, location, and personnel; and second, including such facts helps the researcher recall the whole incident, capture the overall feeling of it, and perhaps recall details that are not in the notes.

Adding Analytic Details

As we will discuss again in Chapter Eight, data collection and analysis are intertwined in anthropology. Analysis begins on the first day of collection. Remember the threefold cycle discussed in Chapter Five: *intuition of whole, specification of parts, and comparison of cases.* This is a continuous process that is revisited each time new data are added. An observation can be thought of as a case, which might add to the specification of new parts (that is, addition of new questions), as well as to the refining of the intuition of the whole (appreciation of new relationships).

When thinking about what she has seen, an anthropologist would ask the following questions:

1. Why did this happen the way that it did?
2. How is it related to my intuition of the problem?
3. What are the elements of it that I do not understand, where do I need to look and what questions do I need to ask in order to fill in that understanding?
4. How is this material related to other observations I have made? What are the similarities and differences, or *patterns* that it illustrates?

As the researcher notes her observations, she will continually ask questions like these, as well as adding hypothetical answers or *hunches* concerning the relevance of the notes to the problem at hand.

One good way of adding analytic details so that they can be easily found in the notes is the *right hand notes, left hand comments* method. One simply keeps all notes of observations on the right hand pages of a notebook, leaving the left hand pages blank for the addition of comments.

INTERVIEWING

Interviews are the second major source of anthropological data. They are used to gather the knowledge, opinions, experience, feelings, and ideas of different actors in the drama of local life. Throughout the research process, starting with the initial design, the researcher will continuously consider:

- whom to interview;
- under what circumstances;
- about what topics;
- using what interview formats;
- with what data recording methods; and,
- with what recruitment strategies.

These decisions are of course interrelated. They are informed by one's sense of problem and question, that is, by a sense of what information is needed, and who might be able to provide it, in what form, and under what circumstances. Very often, these decisions are made on-the-spot during participant observation; they are interviews of opportunity, arising when one finds oneself able to talk to someone who appears to have useful knowledge or interesting opinions. Some of one's best data often come from such situations. As with direct observation, one wants to minimize distortion of the incoming information, promote good rapport, collect a wide variety of knowledge and viewpoints, and keep thorough and accurate records.

Minimizing Distortion

Minimizing the effect of the interviewer on the material (see subsequent section, *Getting the Truth Through Interviews*) entails an effort to make the interview process and setting as close to an ordinary real life situation for the respondent as possible, given the need for privacy and uninterrupted time. If possible, it is usually best to interview someone in his or her own home or other very familiar private place, at a time of their choosing. The situation should be structured like a familiar social meeting, including the local conventions about greeting rituals, gift exchange, polite mood setting conversation, and departing rituals. Symbols (clothes, jewelry, equipment, insignia, etc.) that distinguish between the social status of the interviewer and informant should usually be avoided if possible.

The interview process itself should seek to encourage a relaxed, confident attitude. There are many styles of interviewing, depending on the objective, from highly structured surveys to very spontaneous natural conversation.

Closed-Ended Versus Open-Ended Interviews

Interviews with very specific questions requesting short preprogrammed answers (for example, "yes, no, don't know," or "rate from one to five") are generally called *closed-ended*, in contrast to *open-ended* interviews, which ask the respondent to use his or her own words in answering. Referring back to the naturalistic theory of knowledge, remember that the goal in anthropological interviewing, at least initially, is to capture the meaning of people's perceptions and knowledge in the context of their overall lives. For this purpose, more open-ended and natural ways of interviewing are generally the most valuable.

One particularly useful method is the *open-ended focused interview*. This is a method in which the researcher begins not with a list of specific questions, but with a list of topics about which he or she would like information. Following the natural flow of conversation, and allowing the interviewee considerable freedom in setting the direction, the interviewer asks directive questions as needed in order to get as much knowledge as possible about the topics on the list.

Such an interview usually begins, after the usual greetings and pleasantries, with simple questions such as the interviewee's age, education, marital status, and so on – questions that require little thought, are not likely to stress the interviewee, and set the tone that this is a scientific study.

Following this, the interviewer begins to ask very general, open-ended questions from the list of topics. Listening carefully to the answers, the interviewer then focuses on more specific details needed to fully understand the interviewee's responses.

EXAMPLE: Community Health Interview

(I = interviewer, R = respondent):

I: *I'm interested your ideas about the health problems in this community. Can you tell me about that?*

R: *Sure. There's too much pollution around here. My neighbor has a cough all the time from the pollution. She goes to the herbalist all the time, trying new herbs for the cough, but it doesn't go away. Just the other day I saw her on the bus coming back from town where she went to the pharmacy. Her daughter works at the café across from the district office [in town], so she goes there to see her daughter. Her son is going to school there next year...*

I: *I see. Later I have some more questions about where people shop for medicines. Tell me, what kind of pollution causes these problems? Where does it come from?*

R: *The air is bad. People spray their crops with weed killer. Also, there's too many cars and trucks on this road, it causes a lot of dust. It's gotten so I can't hang my clothes out to dry around here...*

I: *Interesting. Are there other health problems that are caused by this?*

R: *Mostly coughs and colds. I think if you don't get rid of a cough it can go into pneumonia. That happened to old Mrs. Q over here, she lived by herself...*

I: *Who do you think gets these coughs and colds the most?*

R: *Well, I don't know. People who work around here, I guess.*

I: *And are there other kinds of pollution problems too?*

R: *That's the main one, I think.*

I: *Are there other health problems around here besides pollution?*

R: *Well, medicine costs too much, that's certainly a problem.*

I: *Tell me about that.*

R: *(Talks about what it costs to buy medicine, how expensive health insurance is, and how hard it is to make a living here.)*

I: *Okay, any other thoughts about major health problems here?*

R: *(thinking) No, I guess that's about it.*

I: *Okay. You were just talking about money problems people around here have. Can you tell me a bit more about that?*

Note how in the example, the interviewer stayed with open-ended questions, brought the conversation back to the topic at hand, and sought to clarify each of the responses, to fix the respondent's meaning fairly clearly. Note also how the interviewer makes the conversation seem natural, by going to the topic of economics (also on her list of discussion topics) that the respondent had raised, instead of breaking off the flow with a different topic altogether.

The direction of the interview is set jointly by the interviewer and the respondent. This way, the interviewer learns what is uppermost in the respondent's mind. Suppose the interview had started out with a list of health problems from which the respondent was asked to pick the important ones:

I: *Here is a list of common community health problems. Please tell me which of these you think is a problem in this community.*

- *poor sanitation*
- *traffic accidents*
- *poor nutrition*
- *air and water pollution*
- *domestic violence*
- *alcoholism*
- *crime*
- *lack of health knowledge*
- *lack of exercise*
- *lack of good medical care*
- *mental and physical stress*

By this method, the researcher might have diluted the information in several ways. First, she would not have known what the words *health problem* meant to the respondent. Second, she might have put into the respondent's mind the idea of talking about certain things that the respondent had never actually thought about at all. The respondent might never have considered domestic violence to be a health problem, but seeing the list she might think, "Oh, we do have that, I guess it's a health problem," and for that reason she might choose it. The researcher then would put both this choice and the choice of *pollution* in the category of *perceived health problems*, which would have been inaccurate.

There is, however, no perfect way to solve these problems of validity. The nature of human communication is such that we can only approximate knowing what people think. As the philosopher Ludwig Wittgenstein said, "The purpose of language is not to reveal the structure of thought."

Getting Truth Through Interviews

The practice of interviewing people to learn about their knowledge, attitudes, and beliefs is as full of problems as it is common in science, law, education, and journalism. Most cultures have the common sense idea that people have certain knowledge and opinions in their heads, and that we can learn these simply by asking the right questions. But both careful self-reflection and recent psychological science reveals that this view is much too simple. A conversation is far more – and less – than the exchange of what people carry around in their heads.

One obvious challenge to the view that conversation elicits already existing thought comes from the fact that all of us are constantly inventing ideas, deducing opinions, discovering feelings, and perceiving new information every day. In fact, one of the things that makes conversation so pleasurable is that through it, we are constantly discovering or inventing new ways of experiencing life. I might never have thought about the question, "What are the major health problems in my community," but if someone asks me, I can scan my inner store of perceptions and attitudes, and come up with a tentative answer right that minute. Or, I might have given the question a lot of thought, and have a strongly held and complex opinion about it. How would you know which was the case? If you challenge my tentative answer, I might defend it, simply because I don't want to appear ignorant.

But this is only the beginning of the problem of eliciting *true* thoughts. Remember the discussion of *meaning* and *context*, in Chapter Three? Ideas are not stored in our brains like data in little files that can be searched and retrieved like a library catalogue or a computer database. Rather, they are stored as parts of complex systems, more like passages in books. The context in which an idea or symbol is stored affects its meaning for us. For this reason, people often seem to contradict themselves in conversation, without being able to see the contradictions. It is not only possible but common, for example, for someone to simultaneously believe that colds are caused by viruses, and that you should wear warm socks, or say a prayer and light a candle, to avoid getting colds. Socrates, the great Greek philosopher, taught his pupils profound ideas simply by asking them questions in such a way that they could see the hidden implications of what they themselves thought they believed.

Conversation, it turns out, is a creative process by which opinions are formed (often temporarily), knowledge is created, and perceptions are changed. Recall the example in Chapter Four of my relationship with Mrs. Kondo. As the context of our conversations evolved over the months, different *truths* about her situation came to the foreground.

What, then, do we mean by *truth*, or *validity* of interview data? I believe it is this: If we are careful to let people express their everyday ideas, trying not to make them think too much or to compare their thoughts with ours, what people say and do over time in many different situations, exhibits *patterns* of thought, broad habits associated with certain contexts and questions, that give a certain consistency to their actions.

These patterns have some internal consistency, and they differ from person to person according to one's position in society, personality, and needs.

However, these patterns are usually subtle and complex. Different observers, interested in different questions, are likely to see different patterns in what people say. For this reason, the naturalistic theory of knowledge allows us to say we have achieved validity when we have found patterns in our conversations that seem useful to us, and when we can persuade others also that these patterns are useful.

Maintaining Rapport

Maintaining good rapport is also, of course, a way of minimizing the distortion of data. When people feel that they are not being judged by the interviewer or others present, and that their privacy will be respected, they are less likely to "edit" their answers so as to avoid problems or disrespect. Chapter Six, on role taking, contains most of the important suggestions about maintaining rapport with interviewees. Let me just repeat that good rapport is usually built gradually, at the expense of considerable time.

People like to feel that the interviewer is interested in them as personalities, and not simply in their input to the research. People often appreciate time spent chatting in a relaxed way about whatever interests *them*, whether it is part of the study or not. Showing an interest in people's hobbies, family, photographs, home, work, and worries is often a great morale builder. If you are interested in kin groups or families, asking to see photos can be a great icebreaker and a powerful source of information. In many cultures, bringing a small gift as part of one's visit is appreciated, or expected. Whether or not to pay interview subjects in cash depends on local customs, the feelings of the subjects, and the role taken by the researcher. Use your judgment.

A variety of special techniques are needed for dealing with difficult interview topics or particularly shy respondents. Health professionals often have some training and experience in how to talk with patients about death and grief, mental illness, drug and alcohol use, sexual behavior, domestic violence, and other topics that might make a person feel ashamed. Skills at building trust, showing empathy, and establishing a relaxed interview climate are highly valuable. Novice researchers are often quite tense themselves about asking difficult questions, thereby increasing the respondent's anxiety. I find that when I am able to appear calm and confident in asking questions, respondents usually reflect the same attitude and are remarkably open about discussing private things. Often people have been keeping painful feelings and thoughts to themselves for long periods, and feel greatly relieved to be able to express them in a safe setting.

There are also many special techniques for helping people express subtle perceptions, feelings, or personality traits that they are not able to talk about directly – such projective measures and assessment scales as the Rorschach, Thematic Apperception Technique, Myers-Briggs Personality Inventory, various I.Q. and attitude tests, and so on. My advice about using these methods is that they can be useful supplements to straight-forward interviewing once the researcher has developed a thorough personal knowledge of what they actually reveal about people in a particular culture.

Feelings and perceptions about oneself are particularly hard to discuss, partly because people do not want to reveal negative things about themselves, and partly because they do not want to appear vain. In a study I did of mental health among Korean American elderly, I decided to ask people to rate a list of about fifty adjectives, according to which ones they felt described: (a) what they themselves were really like; (b) what they would like to be like; and (c) how they thought other people saw them. This turned out to be extremely useful data, but not because the choice of this or that adjective revealed much. Rather, it turned out that there was a highly consistent set of adjectives that were included in the list of *like me* choices of nearly all the well-adjusted elderly Koreans. People whose choices did not include at least most of this set almost always had serious emotional problems. To explain why this was the case would have taken another research project, for which I did not have the time or money. However, recognizing the pattern helped me a great deal to recognize some people who had problems that were not easy to see at first.

An important part of all interviews is to bring them to a pleasant close, and to request permission to speak to the respondent again at some future time if necessary, even if you think it is unlikely you will need to. People like to feel that there is some continuity in a relationship, and you may actually need to re-interview a given respondent if there are gaps in your understanding, if new questions come up that he or she can answer, or if data somehow get lost.

Keeping Interview Records

We have already discussed the relative advantages of using tape recorders versus taking notes. Each researcher should develop his or her own style in this respect. In general, I do not find that the use of a tape recorder interferes with the quality of interviews if the relationship between researcher and respondent is a good one. People usually forget very quickly that they are being recorded, and things proceed as normal.

Taking notes for interviews can be difficult, because of the need to keep eye contact most of the time with the respondent. My solution is to keep very brief shorthand notes, then go back and write in all the missing material directly after the interview. The same format one uses for observational notes can be used for interview notes. Be sure to write in your notes (whether you are making a recording or not) things that occur that are not strictly part of the interview. When one is closely absorbed in the task of interviewing, important activities going on around it can be completely overlooked and forgotten. Sometimes it is useful to make a back-up recording of interviews, just to check on these unnoticed factors.

Once, having expanded and transcribed my written notes from an interview with a Guatemalan woman in her home, I checked my audio recording to see if I had left anything out. To my amazement, I discovered that throughout the interview she had been arguing with her daughter who was in the background, and I had completely failed to notice this! Instead I had been fully concentrated on understanding her Spanish, taking notes, and planning my next questions.

In addition, there are two habits in keeping interview records that I find very useful. First, always record details of the setting where the interview takes place, its duration, the respondent's appearance, and any unusual details about the situation. These notes should describe the room or other space, including things like noise level, presence of other people, activities going on (including what the respondent is doing, if anything), date and time and weekday, weather and season, the respondent's dress and general appearance (mood, energy level, apparent health, and physical description). Signs of the respondent's attitude toward the interview are also useful. If the interview takes place in the respondent's home, does it appear as though it has been tidied up, or not? Is food or drink served? What about the respondent's dress and demeanor?

Sometimes physical details may indicate the interviewee's state of mind: One of the elderly Japanese American women I interviewed spoke at length of her respect for her long-deceased husband, although there were no photos or other mementos of him to be seen in her home. The second time I visited her, my notes show, a large handsomely framed photo of him had been placed prominently in the living room.

In everyday life, we constantly rely on our semi-conscious intuitions about people and events, and I believe usually with successful results. The second useful habit of interview recording is to make these intuitions conscious and write them down – to always add to the notes of each interview a summary paragraph that describes one's own reactions to it. Did you find it enjoyable, tense, boring, puzzling, depressing, frightening, amusing? Any idea why? Was there anything unusual about it? Did events in your own life, or your health or mood, have an effect on it? Did you find yourself comparing this person with others, and in what ways? Did you get any ideas about the respondent's feelings toward you or the task, or about the openness or guardedness of the answers? If you write these things down immediately after the interview: (a) you will have an accurate record of things that might affect the interpretation of its content, and (b) you will find it far easier to remember other details of the interview once you recapture its mood.

UNOBTRUSIVE MEASURES

Aside from observing the environment and daily life, and talking to people, there are many other sources of information about communities. These *unobtrusive measures* can be used only with care not to violate individuals' rights to privacy. As a matter of course, one should use only those that are open to public use, and even then, only with the permission of the community members. This still might leave a sizeable list of possibilities. Routine records of health-related items such as:

- immunizations, anonymous clinic visits, or disease diagnoses by year, neighborhood, age and gender;
- anonymous police and court records of disputes and arrests by neighborhood, year, and type;
- aggregate data on economic conditions (land and other assets, income, welfare payments, employment rates), education and literacy, business statistics, infrastructure (water, electricity, etc.), environmental conditions, voting behavior, public opinion polls, and so forth.

Reviewing records of such data over time to identify trends may lead to a search for explanations for those trends, which can in turn reveal critical community dynamics that cannot be seen on a short time-scale or learned from polite conversation.

Anthropologist Emma Tarlo set out to study land ownership in a suburb of Delhi, India. Upon examining the relevant government archives and the neighborhood itself, she found dramatic discrepancies both within the archives and between the archives and the physical facts. Explaining these discrepancies led her to many fascinating discoveries about the illegal ways in which land titles were allocated and taxes assessed – discoveries that revealed major hidden dynamics in Delhi politics (Tarlo, 2003).

Comparing such data with regional or national norms can reveal differences that raise important questions about the unique patterns of the local situation, and also suggest the limits of generalizing one's findings.

INDIRECT INDICATORS

Often, things that are difficult or impossible to observe directly can be guessed at by looking at their more obvious effects. These effects are called *indirect indicators*. Before drawing a conclusion from such indicators, try to confirm your guesses by other means also.

EXAMPLE: Vehicles in Thai Village Suggest Rapid Economic Change

I was recently in a remote Thai village, training a group of district hospital workers on how to do community assessment. Walking around the streets, I noticed that there were many motor scooters, nearly all of them very old, and several pickup trucks, all of them brand new. I guessed that the village economy had improved quite recently, and that people were beginning to replace their scooters with trucks thanks to greater wealth. A conversation with hospital personnel confirmed that this was true.

Visible differences between neighborhoods and communities can often reveal differences in social attitudes and behavior. It is simple enough to identify disintegrating neighborhoods by their barred windows and doors, police patrols, gang graffiti, litter, empty lots and buildings, liquor stores and pawn shops, and other warning signs; or wealthy neighborhoods with expensive shops and large well-kept houses.

More subtle signs of neighborhood health and well-being can be read in such things as the number, types, membership, and activities of community organizations; the amount, type, condition, and use of public space; the frequency of various kinds of stores or vendors and the volume of different types of sales (cough medicine, antacids, birth control products, tobacco and alcohol, fruits and vegetables, computer games, cell phone cards, books and magazines, etc.). Recall my earlier vignette about the absence of store signs on a Havana boulevard, and the social implications of that detail.

One data collection skill is to think of what indirect signs might be related to your research question, and how to look for those signs. Another skill is to keep your eyes open for unusual signs you may not understand, and try to find out whether they have any bearing on your problem.

SUMMARY

In anthropology, data collection and analysis are not separate processes, but are intertwined. The day one begins to collect information about a community, one begins to compare the findings to one's intuition about the research question, and to refine the data collection strategy and the question itself.

Data collection usually begins with background research about the study site or population – consulting what is already known about its history, culture, environment, and structure. This background research helps to refine one's intuition of the research problem, and to generate fruitful questions and observations. Throughout data collection, one not only refines one's search for useful information, but one also stays constantly alert for new *incidental* information – unexpected things that might clarify one's questions.

Rapport with the study community is of the highest importance. The researcher must have a plan for maintaining rapport, and must be sensitive to how she is perceived throughout the research.

Interviewing is less a matter of absorbing pre-existing knowledge and opinions than a matter of a dialogue, through which the respondent's view of the topic comes into being. It is important to keep detailed records of conversations, so that the effect of the dialogue itself on the results can be seen and included in the analysis. *Facts* collected in interviews should be checked, whenever possible, against other sources of data, such as direct observation, and unobtrusive and indirect measures.

CHAPTER EIGHT

Analyzing Data

GUIDE TO THIS CHAPTER

In this chapter, I offer some observations about ways of analyzing data that my students and I have found helpful.

Learning to analyze naturalistic anthropological data is like learning a complex intellectual game such as chess or gó, or a craft, like knitting or painting. It is not hard to learn the formal rules, but the rules themselves do not tell you how to play the game or apply the craft skillfully – that takes practice. The early stages of learning can be frustrating, because your results may not be satisfactory. Learning the game of anthropological analysis therefore requires a strong desire to succeed, plus a certain aptitude or skill. One must be able to recognize coherent patterns in complex data, for example.

Also like learning a game or craft, every anthropologist develops a particular *style* of analysis – a way of solving problems using one's own unique perceptions and skills. Toward this end, I suggest that you would do well to study other books on data analysis as well, and to adapt whatever advice is offered to whatever works and feels comfortable to you. Part of the learning process should also be the study of finished ethnographic reports, because they offer examples of how other anthropologists have approached their data. (I believe this is a special problem for nonanthropologists, who may have a different idea of the relationship between data and results than the anthropologist has.) I devote a section of this chapter to the question of how to learn technique from reading anthropology.

Like data collection, data analysis begins on the first day of research. It is a process of making what was at first unclear and intuitive more clear and explicit. In other words, it is a search for regularities and patterns in complex information, guided by experience, models, theories, and intuitions that tell us what kinds of patterns might be useful. We use our everyday skills of pattern recognition. As a pattern begins to emerge, we constantly ask what other observations might improve or weaken our confidence about the usefulness of our intuition, and how we might make those other observations.

This chapter gives examples of methods of analysis, such as content coding and the use of statistics. We also present ways of managing data to make it easier to see patterns, such as the use of diagrams, tables, and lists. Such tools are intermediate steps, and can be revised or discarded as needed.

We also discuss how to read ethnographic texts so that we learn from them what is useful for our own purposes, and how to write results so that they will be persuasive and maximally useful to others.

DATA ANALYSIS USES NATURAL HUMAN SKILLS

I once had the good luck to hear the famous anthropologist Margaret Mead show and discuss the ethnographic films that she and Gregory Bateson made in Bali and New Guinea in the 1930s. During the showing, someone asked her, "How often do you have to see a particular behavior before you realize it is part of the cultural pattern?" Professor Mead said, "We always get that question when we show these films, and I always remember the first time someone asked it. Gregory [Bateson] said, 'How many times? Oh, a few times.' Then he thought a bit and said, 'No. Just once. If you know the cultural pattern, you can tell the first time if the behavior fits or not.'"

This process of looking for useful patterns in a complex field of perceptions is a natural human ability. All of us do it easily, skillfully, and unconsciously every day. Our minds have evolved precisely toward the perfection of this skill. For example, we can often tell immediately if someone we know well is feeling ill or behaving strangely, even if they are trying to conceal the fact. Without being able to say just how we know, we can detect a shift in the overall pattern of the person's behavior that we have come to know intuitively. Likewise, if we are familiar with a certain artist's or composer's work, we can usually recognize an example of it at once, even if we have never seen this example before. We can recognize a well-known face, even if it has grown old, lost its hair, grown a beard, and put on glasses since the last time we saw it.

The same is true of cultural traits. The reason we say culture is *patterned* is because it exhibits the same kind of recognizability that a face or a painting style has. In fact, we can say that much of the work of doing anthropology is the same kind of work as that of getting to know a person or a style of art or music. It is a matter of looking and listening carefully until we have accumulated a considerable store of information, and then letting our innate skill at pattern recognition tell us what the patterns here are.

What makes anthropology different from everyday behavior is, of course, that we try to communicate our learning to other people, instead of just carrying them around in our heads. You might say this makes us different from other people in the sense that an artist or composer is different from one who appreciates art or music. We must be able to express in useful ways to others what we have taught ourselves naturally and intuitively. Let us then focus on this process of making our natural understanding of pattern conscious.

ANALYSIS: MAKING OUR IMPLICIT UNDERSTANDINGS EXPLICIT

Analysis – making our intuitive understandings conscious – is basically a process of *explicitly and consciously* asking and answering questions about our data – questions that clarify and enrich our understanding of the research problem. We are constantly going through our materials – notes, drawings, maps, photos, and materials such as books, articles, news clippings, minutes of meetings, and so on – and asking *how do these facts fit into, or alter, or extend, my intuition of the research problem?*
  In this search, we can distinguish several kinds of questions:

- *Is this part of an important pattern, or is it a unique or trivial finding?* This is largely a *case comparison* question. Let's say in your research you find a case of a person with AIDS who is treated with scorn in the community, while two other patients – one who is blind, and one with arthritis – are treated very kindly. What is causing these reactions? Is there something about the illnesses, or about the status of the patients, or are these reactions about something else altogether – such as the personalities of the victims?
- *Classification questions: What goes with what?* You want to design a health project that people will find important and support. You ask a hundred people in the community what the biggest health problems are, and there are fourteen different popular answers. How can you classify these answers in a way that will tell you the best place to start? Can the answers be grouped into types – such as social, environmental, and economic? Do certain kinds of answers go with certain roles in the community, such as men versus women, elders versus youth, or affluent versus poor?
- *What is missing?* What new observations or comparisons do you need to make in order to understand the relationship between an observation and the research problem? Suppose you want to teach people how to avoid respiratory and gastrointestinal infections.

You find that people keep mentioning *cold* when you talk to them about health and illness. What exactly do they mean by *cold*? (Cold weather? A feeling of coldness in the body? The actual temperature of the body? Lack of warm clothing or bedding?) Are there different types of illness-causing *cold*? How does *cold* cause illness? How does one avoid or treat *cold*? Who believes this explanation and who does not, and why? Is the diagnosis of *cold* part of a coherent pattern of belief about the relationship between health and temperature? Is this a new belief, part of changing patterns in the community, or is it traditional? This is largely a matter of the specification of parts.

- *How do you account for inconsistencies?* You notice that everyone locks their doors in the neighborhood, and many keep aggressive dogs, and some even have guns. You think perhaps people would like to discuss the problem of crime, but instead many tell you that there is no crime here. How do you reconcile these facts? Does the comment that there is no crime mean the people mistrust the police and want to keep them away from the neighborhood? Are they afraid that if they organize against crime, the criminals will cause more trouble for them? Or are they simply so used to the threat of crime that they scarcely even notice their own insecurity?

- *I think I see a pattern: What other questions or observations can I use to test and refine it?* It seems to me that the people in this community do not trust anyone who represents the government or outside authority. At a meeting, a group of them accused the local health post staff of treating them disrespectfully. I have heard them accuse two of the local policemen of taking bribes. Few people participated in a recent school activity. A health department official says they do not follow his instructions. What other observations can I make to test and refine this idea? Are there some officials they trust and others they do not? Do some people in the community trust the government and others not? Who, and why? Can their feelings be changed, and how?

DATA MANAGEMENT

By constantly asking questions like these with your intuition of the research problem in mind, you will begin to extend and refine the intuition. As you solve inconsistencies and fill in the details of incomplete or puzzling findings, you will become more confident that you have found useful answers to research questions.

As you accumulate more and more data, it becomes more difficult to remember all the details of what you have found. At this point, it becomes useful to begin to *manage* your data – to code your notes by subject, to make lists, diagrams and tables, to summarize knowledge in forms that make it easier to see patterns. The arrangement of data in orderly forms also helps in data collection, as it shows where the gaps in one's knowledge are. Again, the tools one selects for data management must be tailored to the needs of the research problem, the setting, and the individual researcher's own style of thinking and working. The following items are only examples of the kinds of data management tools one can use. Textbooks on qualitative data analysis list other management tools. Creative researchers often invent their own.

Kinship Diagrams, or *Genograms*

Information about how people are related to one another by descent or marriage is usually highly useful for several reasons. For one thing, kinship usually plays an important role in how people interact. It tends to be highly culturally patterned, and therefore useful in predicting behavior as well as in identifying anomalies that need to be explained. As with any data management method, what one wants is a simple system of notation that reveals a great deal of information on a single page. A simple way of diagramming kinship, then, is the notation system shown in Figure 8.1.

Symbol	Meaning
△	male
O	female
|	descent
—	siblings
⧄	deceased
=	married
≠	divorced
63△	age

Figure 8.1 Kinship notation chart

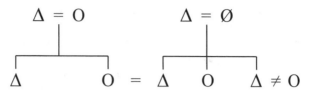

Figure 8.2 Genogram.

A typical kinship chart or *genogram*, then, might look like Figure 8.2, which shows a couple with an unmarried son and a daughter who is married to the son of another couple, the wife of whom is deceased, and who also have an unmarried daughter and second son, who is divorced. Adding names, ages, and other data (for example, health status) to such diagrams is of course a simple matter.

Classification Trees, Organization Charts

You are probably already familiar with organization charts, which show the lines of authority and decision making in businesses and agencies. In an organization chart, the vertical dimension, or the arrow symbol, is usually used to show the direction of authority (generally *top down*), and the horizontal dimension to show separations of function (for example, planning, accounting, sales, production). Some anthropologists use a similar method to show how concepts are related to each other in ascending orders of generality. For example, see Figure 8.3.

Figure 8.3 tells you: (1) that some illnesses, but not all, are caused by supernatural forces; (2) some injuries, but not all, are also supernatural; (3) that all mental illnesses are caused either by witchcraft or spirit

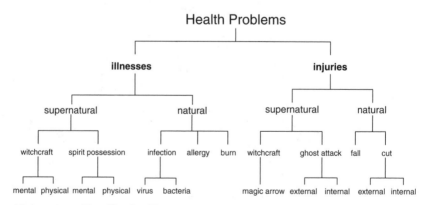

Figure 8.3 Classification Tree.

possession; (4) that witches, spirits, and ghosts can all harm people; and (5) that witches can cause a variety of health problems through a variety of methods. This kind of information might be helpful in discussing causes and cures with members of this culture. Classification trees like this can be built for many kinds of concepts, such as foods, healing techniques, art forms, and games.

Networks and Flow Charts

Diagrams can greatly simplify information about who (individuals, families, or organizations) share what (information, material aid, symbolic gifts, authority) with whom, and how processes work. This kind of summary information can be useful in understanding power and prestige structures, economic activities, and ritual obligations. Sometimes, previously unseen features of social organization emerge from the study of such networks. In its simplest form, the network simply connects individuals with arrows, showing the direction and kind of exchange.

Suppose your interview notes and observations show that certain families cooperate during rice planting season, and others do not. You also notice that this cooperation is sometimes symmetrical (each family helps in the fields of the other), and other times it is not (one family helps, but the help is not returned). You also notice that some, but not all, of the families that cooperate during planting also exchange gifts at New Year's. So you begin to make a diagram of who gives what to whom, as shown in Figure 8.4.

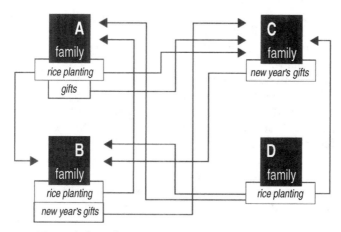

Figure 8.4 Network flow chart.

Looking at this diagram might give you some interesting questions about the relative status of the different families, as well as about the symbolic meaning of collective work and gift giving.

Face Sheets

One method of data management that I find helpful is to summarize, in a systematic and theoretically relevant way, all the data from a particular *case* on a single sheet of paper, as in the example shown in Figure 8.5. A case can be an individual person, a family, a behavioral setting (such as a work place, clinic, public event, school class, etc.), an organization, or a process (such as the diagnosis and treatment of an illness). The purpose is to make it easy to compare different cases, in search of similarities and differences. This is called a *face sheet*.

This face sheet method does several things. First, it reduces the complexity of each case to its most basic and theoretically important elements. Second, it allows the researcher to see an outline of the entire case at a single glance, thereby clarifying relationships among various *variables*, or areas of interest within the case. Third, it serves as a memory enhancer. When one sees the whole case summarized in a single source, , one may recall many previously forgotten details about it. Fourth, it makes it easy to sort cases into groups, according to their similarities and differences, in search of complex patterns. Fifth, it serves as an index to one's complete notes on each case.

Figure 8.5 is an example of a face sheet summary that I made of a lengthy open-ended interview. The interview was part of a study I did which focused on immigration and mental health among Korean-American elderly in San Francisco in the 1980s. Comparing the face sheets of sixty interviews allowed me to rate individual interviewees as *well-adjusted* or *having adjustment problems*. By comparing these two classes of people, I could see: (a) that there were certain common sources of stress that seriously interfered with adjustment; and (b) that the well-adjusted people fell into four different *styles of coping*.

Looking at this example, first note the names of the categories in which I chose to summarize the interview data. These categories were partly derived from my first intuition about what would be important in determining the elderly Koreans' mental health, but they were also in part derived from my study of the interview data as is came in.

The first category is that of *demographic data* – basic facts such as age, gender, education, date of immigration, and occupation. (Since many immigrants had different jobs in Korea and in the United States, I listed both of these.) Such facts generally have an overwhelming influence on

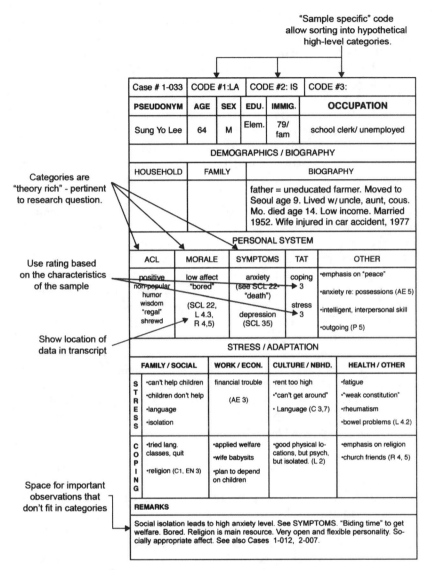

Figure 8.5 Face sheet.

the life of every human being in one way or another, so it simply makes sense to keep them in the summary.

The second category is that of *biographical data* – the structure of the person's household, the structure of their extended family, and unusual events in the individual's life history.

The third category is called the *personal system*. In this study I was interested in mental health. My intuition suggested that I could measure this partly by asking about people's morale, partly by understanding their sense of self-worth, and partly on a scale of psychiatric symptoms. In addition, I wanted to know what was unique about each individual personality, and I included the category *Other* to record unusual features that did not fit anywhere else. I also used this section to rate each case according to an *ipsative* (that means the scores were developed from the data at hand and are not applicable to other samples) five-point scale for stress level and coping ability. The section labeled *ACL* summarizes the results of an Adjective Check List I administered to measure self-concept.

The fourth category is that of *stress and adaptation*. Although my initial intuition suggested that these things would be important to measure, the category expanded as I looked at the data. I could see that people's relationships with their family, their work and economic situation, their ethnic group (other Koreans in the area) and neighborhood were all critically important. Here I also included a section on what their health problems were, and how they dealt with those problems.

Note the final section, called *Remarks*. Every face sheet should have a space for features of the case that do not fit neatly into any of the categories, but one's intuitive understanding of the case suggests are important enough to be included in the summary. These comments often generate new insights, and can lead to extensive reanalysis of the data.

Somewhere on the face sheet (here it is at the top), there should be a place for codes. In the process of comparing cases, we generate hypotheses about what goes with what – what patterns we are seeing. We classify cases according to pattern configurations or types, we name these types, and we record which type each case belongs to. In this study, I found that acculturation levels, social supports, personality, and religious/philosophical beliefs together formed complex styles of living that helped to explain people's adaptation or lack of it.

Using the face sheets from the study illustrated here, I was able to create summary profiles of the entire sample, showing the means and distributions for all values – age, gender, immigration date, education, family size, number of children, and ratings on stress and coping.

Looking at the entries on the face sheet in Figure 8.5, notice several things.

First, kinship diagrams can be used in the Family and Household boxes to show all sorts of useful information (e.g., one can mark with an asterisk members of the subject's family in the United States). This may be critical information, indicating many things about the subject's relations with kin, the family's immigration history, and so on.

Second, notice the kinds of incidents that are mentioned in the *Biographical* section. In this case, a highly stressful incident (wife's car accident) that emerged from his biography was used as an example of how this person perceives and responds to stress. In the *Personal System – Other* category, we note that his interview showed unusually high anxiety about money and luxuries, and noted his high intelligence and outgoing personality. In the *Remarks* section, we note his relative social isolation, his religiosity, and the fact that the interviewer reacted to him as an unusually flexible personality.

Third, notice that there are numbers in parentheses next to many of the entries. These *numbers indicate where in the raw interview one can find the data supporting the comment.* This is extremely important, for several reasons. For one, the researcher is likely to forget exactly why this rating or comment was given, and might need to refer to the raw data to recall. For another thing, if one is rating the cases on a particular value (let us say *anxiety*, for example), it is highly useful to be able to refer directly to the raw data, to confirm one's ratings. Finally, in writing up the data, it is highly useful to be able to insert quotes from the interviews themselves to illustrate for the reader how the ratings were made.

Fourth, notice the numbers in circles in the *TAT* category (which indicates a structured personality test). These are *ipsative ratings*, or ratings I developed based on the sample itself, placing him in a category with certain other respondents who showed the same levels of stress and coping, based on this test.

HOW TO TREAT DATA MANAGEMENT TOOLS

Something to keep in mind in making and using all of these data management tools is that one's first attempts are not likely to represent accurately the final analysis of the data. Rather, data management tools are tentative, flexible, and disposable. One way to think about them is to compare them to the sketches than an artist uses in the process of creating a painting. The artist wants to experiment with different colors, figures, perspectives, light and shadow, application techniques, and compositions. In the process, she may make and discard many sketches, or modify some sketches many times, before beginning the final canvas. At any time during the data analysis process, (which, remember, begins on the first day of data collection) one might have an insight or discover an unsuspected principle that changes the whole research project. Remember the example in Chapter Five about the researcher who set out to study social engagement, and ended up studying attitudes toward death.

In keeping with this principle of their tentative nature, it is important not to give data management tools too much authority. When we see our data neatly laid out in a table or a diagram, it is tempting to think that this schematic actually represents some objective reality, and to forget that we made this representation up ourselves.

As I have said, these are only a few of the tools you can use to increase your power to manipulate data. You can also make lists and tables of all kinds, so that you can compare at a glance things like family size, income, health history, and hundreds of other things.

ANALYZING RAW DATA: CONTENT CODING

Participant observation often involves participating in everyday conversations and watching everyday activities. This gives us a good idea of what the typical beliefs and behaviors in a community are, but often, especially at the beginning of the study, it leaves us with pages and pages of notes whose significance is not clear. One common way to discover subtle behavior patterns is to simply go through these notes and code them – make notations of what subjects are discussed, who is present, what ideas are expressed, and the background features of the action. If one suspects there is a subtle relationship among two or more coded details, one can then abstract them from the narrative for a closer look.

EXAMPLE: Japan Town: Sports Mark Important Social Distinctions

During my study of Japanese Americans in San Francisco, I gradually learned that there was a fair amount of competition among various groups in the community. People would say that a certain person was "not in our circle," or "not a member of our group." This surprised me, because the community was small, and had a reputation for being peaceful and united. It was hard to understand what formed the basis of this competition. I began to code the terms in the data that were associated with competition, terms describing contests, political rivalries, generational rivalries, and disagreements about matters of community concern. Among other things, I discovered that sports played a very important symbolic role in the community. Having discovered this, I began to ask people systematically about their sports participation, their favorite teams, and so on. Virtually everyone between the ages of ten and sixty either belonged to a Japanese American sports team (most commonly basketball, sometimes softball) or was an avid supporter of a team. Teams, in turn, were sponsored by churches and temples, voluntary organizations (such as Boy Scouts), and businesses.

So important was involvement in sports that those who did not participate were sometimes seen as "outside the community" as a whole. Crossing over from one sports team to another was seen as a serious breach of loyalty. Loyalties created major social barriers between groups in this small community. In one instance, a Japanese-American Christian church had to close due to dwindling finances. Rather than merge with a nearby Japanese-American church of the same denomination, they chose to honor their old team rivalry and merge with an African-American church.

Attention to content coding of raw data has produced many other interesting results in all of my studies. When I was studying aging in the Ozark Mountains of Missouri, I coded all references to city life. I learned this way that there was a strong symbolic opposition in country people's minds between city life and country life, which explained a great deal about their behavior. The city was almost universally seen as a lonely place far from kin and community, where a person's needs were not considered, values were not respected, and people in general were simply unfriendly. City people worshipped money, and their way of living was somewhat sinful and shallow. The country, by contrast, was a place where an individual's character and social connections meant more than money or success, and where a man or woman could live an honest and noble life, even in poverty. Country people would often try to "make a go of it" in the city but give up after a few years and return, penniless and homesick, to live lives that seemed to me materially harsh and uncomfortable.

Anthropology, as we have said, seeks to reveal patterns implicit in the way of life under study, rather than to impose our own theoretical models on behavior. Accordingly, we often try to use the words and concepts of the people we are studying as guides to the structures we seek. Probably the most common way to do this is by *coding raw data* according to important concepts that appear in our community members' speech. Sometimes these concepts are unique to the people we are studying, and sometimes they are familiar ideas in cultures around the world, but we want to understand the unique way they are related to other concepts in our study community.

The simplest way to code raw data for content is to simply make marginal notes on data transcripts, and keep an index of the page numbers where the codes appear. Ordinary word processing makes this a fairly easy task. In addition, there are various computer software programs, called annotation aid programs, that serve this purpose. *Atlas-ti* and *Nudist* are two commercial annotation aid programs. Some of my colleagues use them, but I myself prefer hand annotating.

Once a new concept has been identified this way as potentially important, the researcher often wants to systematically collect further information about it, as I did with sports teams in the *Japan Town* example, and with city life as seen from the Ozarks. One thing these examples show,

I believe, is that we cannot always guess at the beginning of a research project where we will find the most useful answers to our problems. This is precisely why the research enterprise must remain open to discovery at every step.

USING STATISTICS

Once the researcher has developed a fairly thorough holistic sense of community life, statistics can also be used to suggest the presence of patterns. If correlations are found between statistical measurements, the anthropologist never automatically infers a simple causal relationship, but uses the correlation to inform new observations and questions.

EXAMPLE: Crime Reports and Housing Density Seem Related. Why?

In Chapter Seven, I gave the example of two adjacent neighborhoods, one in which there was a high degree of community integration and a low crime rate, the other in which the opposite conditions prevailed. If one looks at the statistics describing the two neighborhoods, one finds that population density and police actions in the "unhealthy" community are both significantly higher than in the "healthy" one. From this it would be simple to conclude that high-density housing causes crime. But this would be a misleading conclusion. First, one must understand the relationship between actual crime and police response. One reason there are fewer police actions in the "healthy" community may be that the residents feel safer, and are therefore less likely to call the police if they see something unusual. Another reason may be that the police themselves are more suspicious of people in the "unhealthy" community, and more likely to cruise its streets and make arrests. There is even a possibility that this police behavior alienates the young men in the "unhealthy" community, motivating them to break the law. Next, one must understand the relationship between housing density and social organization. The low density of the housing in the "healthy" community has probably been caused by the strong social organization there, not the other way around. City officials are unable to change the zoning laws there to permit high-density housing, because the residents join together to oppose such changes every time they are proposed. In short, without knowing the histories and daily lives of the two neighborhoods, one is ill prepared to interpret the intriguing statistics.

I have criticized positivist social science for using statistics without sufficient attention to the contexts and meanings of the variables being measured. The result is often that the true meaning of statistical associations is missed. However, much of the data collected in anthropological research can be quantified and subjected to statistical analysis. It is often helpful to do so, *provided that the local meaning and context of measured variables is understood.*

HOW TO READ AND LISTEN TO ANTHROPOLOGY

There are many reasons to read the published work, or listen to the lectures, of other anthropologists. It helps to learn what theories and points of view have been developed that you might draw upon. It improves your understanding of a particular research topic, such as a geographic area or a type of social problem. It allows you to understand various research techniques and their results. And of course it can be a great source of entertainment as well. (And by the way, meeting with other anthropologists and talking informally with them is often an even more efficient way of learning the same kinds of things.)

Here I want to discuss two particular reasons for anthropological researchers to read or hear others' work: (1) to enrich knowledge of the context of your own research; and (2) to refine your technical skills by observing the techniques of others.

Reading for Context

No matter what research methods you use, an important part of understanding the material you collect is to read or listen and understand what other social scientists have written that may be relevant to your problem. Suppose you are studying drug use in an urban Mexican community. At a minimum, you would want to study published work on the following issues:

- the history, ecology, and ethnology of Mexican cities, especially of this particular locale and city;
- the ethnology of the rural areas whose people migrate to this city;
- the politics, economics, culture, and history of drug use in Mexico, with special reference to the drugs you are finding;
- crime, especially narcotics trafficking, and the role and practices of the police in Mexico;
- Mexican youth in general;
- the Mexican health care system as it affects drug users;
- research on similar issues from other societies; and,
- the theories and research perspectives that have been used in seeking to understand such things, and with what results.

Reading in each of these areas will enrich your intuition of the particular problem you are studying, and point out what kinds of questions to ask and things to observe to fill in the gaps in your knowledge. For example, how have immigration patterns affected employment, income, education, and drug use in this city? How are these things different in other cities, or in other countries? How do Mexican youth in other areas, urban and rural, interact with drugs, and why? How do police policies help or hinder in solving the drug problem, and what accounts for those policies? Do the models that have been applied to the understanding of drug use in other populations (counterculture, *anomie*, substitute consumerism, etc.) seem to fit this one, or not?

Reading and Listening for Technique

There are many different kinds of anthropological products, from basic descriptions of field work, to theoretical analyses of a particular culture or phenomenon, to reviews and critiques of another author's work or a whole field of study, to purely theoretical arguments. For ethnographic research methods, reports of field work, and theoretical analyses and critiques of ethnographic studies are the most useful, so I will be referring mainly these types of works.

As we will discuss a little later (see *Writing the Results*) a good ethnographic report or analysis should indicate what theoretical perspective the author is using, and describe how the ethnographer actually worked – what kinds of data she collected and how, where, from whom, and over what periods of time. A brief history of the data collection process can be extremely useful, but few ethnographers actually offer this.

The first principle of reading or listening in order to learn technique, is to keep your own intuition in mind, and constantly compare what is being offered to what you already think about the cases under discussion. Notice that this is very different from accepting anyone else's analysis of anything as final or somehow superior to your own. Some questions you might ask include the following:

1. Do the data differ from what you would expect? If so, why?
2. If there are surprises, are they unique to the situation, or has the author uncovered general features of the phenomenon that had been overlooked by others?
3. What differences are there, if any, between the kinds of questions the author asked, and what you would have asked? How do his questions and yours relate to the intuitions that each of you has?
4. What about the theoretical orientation? Is it similar to yours, or different?
5. Might the author's data, or insights about the data, be applicable to your own research problem or not, and why?
6. How is your intuition of your own research problem changed by what you have heard or read?

Another question to ask is what are the practical results or possible applications of this particular work? (Don't forget the section on the *Idea of Usefulness* in Chapter Three.) Practical results can mean a better theory, as well as a healthier community or a more convincing political argument. So, you might also ask some additional questions, such as:

7. Does this work address, even remotely, your practical concerns?
8. What do the author's practical concerns (stated or unstated) seem to be, and does this analysis seem to fit those?
9. If there are practical differences between you and the author, how would you modify his approach so that the results fit your aims better?

WRITING THE RESULTS

Just as there is no single best way to gather or analyze anthropological data, there is no single ideal way to write the results. In this section I first present what I understand to be the standards of good ethnographic writing; then I discuss some of the uses of ethnographic reports, and the need to match writing style to use.

Good ethnographic writing should:

- persuade the audience that the writer did a competent job of collecting and analyzing her data and understanding her results;
- reveal enough about the research process so that the reader can roughly understand the relationship of the findings to the raw material of community life from which they were drawn;
- use concepts and language that are familiar and understandable to the audience; and,
- address issues and problems that the audience finds useful.

Persuasion

Very few science teachers ever use the word *persuasion* when they talk about doing science. The myth among scientists is that there is only one truth, and that the *weight of evidence* is supposed to lead everyone eventually to that one truth. It is an idea that has a parallel in economics – the best product for the best price is supposed to eventually drive all other products out of the market. In reality, science seldom works exactly this way, especially when dealing with complex problems. Often there is more than one way to understand the data at hand, and each analyst must try to make the best case possible for his or her interpretation by emphasizing the importance of the problems it solves, and de-emphasizing those on which it is weaker. There is nothing dishonest about this, once we accept the naturalistic theory of knowledge – that *truth* is essentially a matter of usefulness.

Transparency

It is quite common in social science writing for the author to assume that all of his or her colleagues use more or less the same techniques, and that it is not necessary to say much about his methods, except perhaps to mention roughly where he worked, when and for how long, how many people he talked to, of what types, and a few other general facts.

Actually, anthropological writing is far more useful if the writer describes what he or she did in some detail, and how it felt. The reader should able to imagine accompanying the ethnographer in her daily work, see the frustrations that she is dealing with, learn the emotions she felt as she encountered the people and events of her study, and above all, learn how the researcher's thinking evolved over the course of the study. With such information in hand, it is much easier for the reader to tell where his viewpoints and judgments coincide with those of the author, and where they diverge. The effect of this is to improve the usefulness of the reporting.

Language

Like all professions, anthropology has developed its own professional language or jargon, a language that uses shortcuts to communicate ideas that are widely known. Also, like all professions, anthropology is subject to intellectual fads. At any given time, a particular group of theories, authors, or analytic problems tends to dominate the thinking of scholars, while other useful viewpoints drop out of favor.

Both these trends have a certain usefulness. Using jargon does make communication easier among specialists. Following fads does encourage scholars to learn new ideas and think about problems in new ways. In my view, however, health workers who are not primarily professional anthropologists do not benefit much from either jargon or fashion-consciousness. Rather, if they try to imitate the way their professional anthropologist contemporaries write, they simply suffer from their drawbacks – failing to communicate clearly with many who might use their ideas.

Usefulness

Keeping in mind that we are using a very broad definition of usefulness, the idea that anthropological writing should be useful might sound too obvious to need comment. I mention it in order to focus attention on the fact that scholars are often tempted to sacrifice practical usefulness in the interest of something else, namely professional prestige. As I mentioned in the earlier discussion of language, professions are communities of scholars with a shared culture. This culture, like any other, includes rules (usually unspoken) about what kind of work is most praiseworthy. Often, this means work that attracts the attention of the most prestigious journals and thinkers in the profession. This, in turn, depends to some extent on the methods, subject matter, and concepts embodied in one's published work.

Up to a point, professionalism itself can be defined as the ability to identify and reproduce the most successful formulae for recognition. Only occasionally does a new work appear that is both novel and persuasive enough to distract the attention of the profession's leaders and confer high prestige on the author. In order to counterbalance this tendency, I encourage you to stay focused on the questions of who might find your work practically useful, and how; and to allow these questions to dominate the way you write.

SUMMARY

Data analysis in anthropological research accompanies and guides data collection. There is no prescribed formula or set of procedures for analysis; it is for the most part simply the careful and systematic recognition and recording of complex patterns of behavior – an ability all human beings use in their everyday lives.

Data analysis is greatly aided by the use of data management tools, such as lists, tables, flow diagrams, genograms, classification trees, and face sheets. These tools simplify and clarify relationships among observations. In addition to the standard ones discussed in this chapter, researchers can and should use their imaginations to create tools that best make sense of their own data.

Often, the adaptation of techniques from positivist or quantitative research also helps analyze descriptive data. Coding rules can be developed for the content analysis of texts. All sorts of factors can be quantified, such as age, gender, health status, income, property, time allocation, church membership, or the size of social networks. Co-variation among such numbers can often raise questions that can lead to the discovery of patterns.

A great deal can be learned about anthropological data analysis from reading published studies and visualizing how the researcher used raw data to reveal patterns and construct explanations.

Writing research results is largely a matter of persuading readers that one's work is useful, and that it has been done systematically and thoroughly. In other words, the researcher must be careful to make clear what the research activity was like, and how the findings were derived from the raw data.

CHAPTER NINE

The Theory of Needs

GUIDE TO THIS CHAPTER

In Chapter Three I mentioned the role of theory in naturalistic research. I said that theories are often important in helping us construct our original intuition of our research problem. A good theory helps us decide where to begin to look to fill out the parts of our intuition and what kinds of cases we need to compare to ground our intuition in the real community. In the process of doing naturalistic research, we extend, refine, and modify our theories, and occasionally come up with new ones.

In this chapter, I offer a theory of health-related behavior that I believe can serve as a useful starting point for doing health anthropology. The *Theory of Needs* provides researchers with material around which to build intuitions about many of the kinds of problems community health workers commonly face – problems such as identifying the barriers to health and healthy behavior that belong to a shared way of life, motivating people to confront those barriers, and making decisions about health interventions that will preserve the healthy aspects of existing cultural systems. Together with the *Theory of Hope* (Chapter Ten), the theory of needs also suggests ways of building community capacity for healthy change.

It is well known that health behavior and health knowledge are related, but the way they are related is not simple or well understood. In this chapter you will learn a new way of thinking about this relationship. Health is only one of many needs, and behaviors can be understood as strategies for balancing these needs – strategies that are in turn adapted to the culture and environment of the individual and the community.

The theory of needs is not something new that I invented myself. It is the result of interaction between existing theories of human behavior, my own research experience, and the research results of others. In keeping with the naturalistic theory of knowledge, I do not claim that this theory is the only, or best, theory of human needs, or even necessarily the best one for health researchers. Every researcher should judge for herself how useful it is.

EXISTING MODEL OF COMMUNITY HEALTH PRACTICE (CHP)

Professional training programs exist in Family and Community Medicine, Public Health, and Community Health Systems Nursing. There are academic programs in Social Medicine. We see the terms *community oriented* and *community based* nursing, medicine, or health care. What are the basic ideas that underlie attempts to address health at a community level – what I will simply call collectively *community health practice*, or CHP for short? There is no generally accepted way for health professionals to approach the health of communities, but most common approaches share certain ways of looking at the two terms, *health* and *community*, which in turn imply an implicit view of human nature and social behavior.

The Concept of *Health*

The unifying theme of community health practice is the idea that ill-health is seen not simply as the result of biological forces, but also as the result of the social, cultural, physical, economic, and political environments which people share as members of communities. Work aimed at improving the health consequences of these environments should have the effect of reducing the risks of ill-health for all those who share them. This in turn should reduce disease and suffering at a cost well below that of the treatment of active illness.

As part of this model, it is generally assumed that health, or at least freedom from disease, is, like human life itself, universally valued, a desired goal of both individuals and communities, and a powerful motive in behavior. It is assumed that if people understand what behaviors lead to good and bad health, and if they have a choice, they will always choose the former, other things being equal. These assumptions are an important feature of the CHP model; it requires the active interest and participation of the recipient communities in order to be effective.

Another important feature of existing CHP models is the definition of health. Some formal definitions by CHP advocates go beyond just the absence of physical and psychological abnormality, and include complete social and spiritual well-being (WHO/UNICEF, 1978). However, in practice, CHP interventions are generally aimed at reducing identifiable causes of physical disease. This is attempted either directly, for example by prescribing diet and exercise, or indirectly, by encouraging people to think about their health more and care for themselves better. This emphasis on physical disease is understandable, given the fact that most CHP programs have little money and have trouble developing ways to solve very complex barriers to well-being. However, I will later argue that focusing solely on the physical side of illness is neither wise nor necessary.

The Concept of *Community*

For our purposes here, a *community* is simply a group of people who share certain problems in common, and who agree to work together to solve those problems. Usually, such a group will have one or both of the following characteristics: (a) its members live close together, as in a village or urban neighborhood; and, (b) they recognize each other as being of the same culture, race, religion, or social class, or as sharing a common history. People who share these characteristics are most likely to recognize each other as possible friends and allies. Such groups are also likely to share common problems. Such health factors as air and water quality, housing quality, climate, transportation, health care, employment, and rates of crime and substance abuse affect geographic areas. Such factors as food preferences, life-styles, kinship and household structure, social resources (cooperation and conflict), and discrimination in jobs, housing and legal rights tend to be shared by people who share cultural background.

It is important to notice two things about our definition of community. First, the word community is often used to mean something other than this. In public health it is an everyday term, often referring to the people in a geographical district, without considering whether they think of themselves as neighbors, or have any interest in cooperating about anything. Second, our definition is quite elastic and changeable. The particular group of people who cooperate to solve common problems is likely to change over time, so that the specific individuals who together formed the community in July might be quite different from those who were included in January.

The Goals and Limitations of the CHP Model

It is understood by community health practitioners that the means to good physical and mental health – good food, water, housing, and sanitation; education; low risk work and living environments; rest and leisure; access to care and treatment – are often in short supply. Who gets access to them is often a matter of wealth and power as much as need. We know there are relative winners and losers in the competition for the means to good health. One of the goals of public health is to help the losers achieve a certain minimum standard of health by helping them get access to the things they need.

Given these goals, core activities of community health practice are the measurement of community health needs, and the design of projects to correct these needs. Importantly, *needs* are generally defined in terms of high rates of shared conditions that result in high rates of diagnosed disease – lack of knowledge, sanitation, nutrition, or services, or prevalence of risky behaviors. Action projects might be narrowly addressed to specific problems, such as exercise and nutrition classes to reduce rates of hypertension, or they might be more systemic, such as giving new primary health care services, or even introducing economic skills to reduce poverty.

Such efforts are often made difficult by several factors: (a) lack of public funds needed to properly and thoroughly plan and carry them out; (b) unwillingness of community members to cooperate, or active opposition by some people; (c) simple ineffectiveness of the plan, due to the complexity of the problem; (d) lack of useful information about the effectiveness of the plan; (e) rapid changes in the cultural, economic, or physical environment that undercut the importance or effectiveness of the work. These problems are interrelated. To continue getting the money and cooperation needed, a project must show rapid and clear progress. It does not seem to be sufficient if there is indirect evidence that CHP is effective as a general way of improving public health.[1]

I believe that the problems faced by the CHP model, and the others I discuss, result from a working definition of health that is still too narrow to produce large, sustainable results. Even though CHP is much broader than the disease model of the clinical sciences, it needs to include even more information. Specifically, the standard CHP model: (a) fails to explain how health is systematically related to other basic human needs; and, (b) fails to think of communities within a wider historical perspective. The result is that health interventions often fail because:

- the competition for attention and resources exerted by other human needs has not been carefully considered; and,
- much more general historical distortions in collective life, of which rates of illness are but a symptom, have not been considered.

These two different limitations of the existing CHP way of thinking turn out to be closely related, and to share a common solution – namely, to view human communities as people meeting needs in patterned context. In

---

[1] Centralized political systems, like China and Cuba, are an exception, and have achieved dramatic success with community health practices. This underscores the upcoming argument about motivation for change.

the section that follows I explain what this means, how it is different from the existing CHP model, and how it promises a more effective approach to community health. For brevity, I will call this the *needs/context model*.

A MORE EFFECTIVE MODEL: PEOPLE MEETING NEEDS IN PATTERNED CONTEXT

To understand health at the community level, anthropology looks not only at measurable rates of ill health and their causes, but at the way health and illness fit into the whole way of life. Members of a community usually share attitudes about what it means to be healthy, and what kinds of behaviors make for a "healthy" person. Some of these attitudes may be very different from those of a health professional, and the differences need to be understood if professionals and communities are to work together.

EXAMPLE: Heart Disease in the Coalfields

The public health department in an area of Australia known as the Coalfields noticed that hypertension and heart disease were major problems there. The population was mostly coal miners and their families, who had little education and who had led hard lives on account of poverty, poor health care, and a low quality of work and living environment. The public health department began a program to educate the people about the causes and effects of heart disease and stroke, and to offer programs of exercise and nutrition. Anthropologists were hired to monitor the program.

After a couple of years, it was found that rates of illness had not changed, but that people were on the whole living longer anyway. The anthropologists explained how this had happened. The residents of Coalfields had a long history of mistreatment by the government, they felt, and they had developed a strong mistrust of all local officials. They also had developed great pride in their toughness and independence, and the way they worked together as neighbors and helped each other. Once they realized that too many people were dying of heart attacks and strokes, they developed their own volunteer ambulance service, in order to get victims to the hospital quickly if they had the symptoms of those illnesses. As a result, many fewer people died of an acute episode (Higginbotham et al., 2001).

Meeting Needs

First, the term *people meeting needs* makes us think about how people are always actively guiding their own lives by making choices themselves. Most CHP advocates would agree with this, and ask, "How is this different from the way we think?" The answer is as follows:

CHP puts attention on the world in which people live as an objective reality. It is a positivistic point of view. According to this view, people are thought of most of the time as reacting to their environment and their own (or their loved ones') health. CHP also assumes that everyone wants to be healthy, and that the choices they make will tend to be healthy choices if people have correct information about their environment and their bodies. However (the CHP thinking goes), people often make health mistakes because they lack the needed information about their environment and their health.

The CHP view of human behavior, in other words, is too simple. It assumes that, aside from a desire for health, and a tendency to react more or less rationally to circumstances, we do not need to know much about human nature. In short, people are seen reacting predictably to an objective situation, not as strategists who actively construct and manipulate their situation to satisfy a whole complex list of wants. I call this the *deterministic model*. The deterministic model looks for missing or incorrect resources or opportunities, an objective situation whose correction will lead to better health. One simply needs to provide the missing knowledge, services, environmental controls, foods, attitudes, and activities. Hypertension is rampant because the people do not know its symptoms, long-term consequences, or causes. People suffer asthma because they cannot afford to live in areas with clean air and good housing.

By contrast, the *needs/context model*, in viewing people as active agents meeting their needs, considers the environment to be in part the result of their purposeful actions. Hypertension is rampant because what people eat, how and where they work, and what they do in their leisure time are part of an integrated life-style that carries great symbolic meaning and confers status and intimacy. Asthma is only one of many diseases people suffer because there are many aspects of their life-style they could not pursue in a healthier location, and they have found that the struggle for health in a hostile environment often robs them of what little well-being their lives afford

Notice two things about this needs/context view of behavior. First, it leads to quite different strategies of work than the deterministic model. Second, in order to apply it, one must begin with a general theory of human needs, in which health is not the only, or even the most important, goal of life-constructing action. I will return to the theory of needs later.

Patterned Context

There is no fixed relationship between human needs and health or illness. Rather, the relationship arises out of the way people in communities organize their lives and construct locally acceptable strategies for getting their needs met. The way people seek respect, for example, will differ greatly from place to place, depending on the local view of what behaviors are admirable, and what resources are available to achieve status. These differences are intelligible only within the overall pattern of the local way of life.

EXAMPLE: Meratus: Birth Control, Fertility, and Respect

Anthropologist Anna Tsing studied a tribal people called the Meratus, living in the mountains of Indonesia. The national government wanted all tribal people to limit the number of children they had, so they had health workers introduce birth control pills to the Meratus villages. The result was that certain men in each village, men who had political ambitions, volunteered to carry out the birth control program. These men then told the rest of the people that these pills would cure disease, and kept the pills in their houses to dole out to those who were sick. Although this response was puzzling to the health authorities, it was quite predictable to one who knew the Meratus culture, for several reasons. For one thing, women there are very subordinate to men, and men gain prestige and power by having lots of children. They are aware that sometimes women resist producing and raising endless babies, but the idea that anyone would want fewer children is one that simply makes no sense to them. For another thing, the government is seen in these villages as a dangerous alien power. Men gain prestige in their villages if they can keep the government away. By pretending to accept the health workers' explanations and accepting the pills, the more ambitious men hoped they would seem powerful and effective, and thereby defeat their political rivals (Tsing, 1993).

Context, Meaning, and Change

The second feature of the needs/context model is its approach to the relationship between health-related behavior and the context in which it occurs. Human actions that influence health cannot be viewed in isolation. One has to understand them in the light of their meaning and purpose for the people who perform them. This meaning and purpose, as we saw in Chapters Three and Four, differs according to the whole system of habits and expectations that surround it. This is pure anthropology, the idea that behavior is determined by a complex interaction of surrounding material facts (physical and social environment, biology, etc.) and the actors' distinct and equally complex, culturally- and biographically-influenced understanding of these facts, and their import for the satisfaction of their own needs.

In its more sophisticated forms, CHP recognizes the importance of context and interpretation. It is widely seen as good practice to assess local cultural understandings and habits regarding a particular health problem, and to study the impact of a particular intervention on the community's way of life, and to shape one's intervention to account for these. Two important things, however, are usually missing in CHP thinking about contexts.

One is a sense of the complex patterning of cultural understandings – of the human habit, greatly influenced by language, of weaving meanings together into interlocking systems whose integrity and continuity limit and structure the kinds of changes that are possible. If the pattern is not there, things do not make sense, and people will shun what does not make sense. Not only is pattern compatibility necessary for meeting basic needs, but the desire for meaning – for the experience of the pattern's integrity – is itself a basic need.

In the following example, members of a low-status African American community had their own shared understanding – an understanding rich with irony – of how they were viewed by white outsiders. They used the lack of respect and understanding they felt directed against them to strengthen their own sense of self-worth as a community.

EXAMPLE: Black Participation in a Predominantly White Conference

In the working class urban African American community where I work, people are accustomed to being excluded from the leadership of White dominated institutions that exist, in part, to help them, such as local, state, and national public health organizations. As a rule, they do not even expect to be consulted by such organizations about what their community needs. Recently, however, some leaders of such authorities have begun to realize that their projects in such communities are failing because they do not understand how the residents themselves think about things like health, justice, and respect. The leaders of a national organization invited our community to send three residents to a large national conference to teach the delegates a few things about the local point of view. Aterward, I was privileged to be at a meeting in the community where these local delegates described their experience.

All three local delegates were low-income women, and all of them were long-term activists who knew the community and its political environment well, and had developed considerable leadership skills. As they understood it (and to some extent they were undoubtedly correct), their job at the national conference was to represent what it meant to be Black and working class. At the community meeting, to howls of laughter, they demonstrated how they had talked and walked and partied, showing their quaint accents and uncultured ways, exaggerating the very behaviors they believed distinguished them from the White majority at the conference. In the end, they said, "They loved us!" They had enacted their understanding of the pattern of race relations – a pattern in which any attempt to seem equal, or intellectually knowledgeable, or worthy of respect on the same terms as the professionals present, would have been rejected. They had, in effect, interpreted the honor of participating in this conference as a confirmation of their cultural beliefs about race relations.

The White delegates at the national conference, for their part, were required by their cultural values to show respect and appreciation for whatever our delegates offered. Did they learn anything useful about how the community works? I have my doubts.

The other missing element is a sense of the process of accommodation by which cultural patterns adapt to new information. If culture were not flexible, it would not work; but this flexibility itself follows patterns – it is not random or unlimited.

Beginning, then, with the idea of cultural patterning: One way to understand this concept is to focus on the fact that Western biomedical science is itself a complex, well-integrated pattern of understanding about health and disease. Those trained exclusively in it cannot see the value of unfamiliar practices without understanding a good deal about the world view of the people that practice them; that is, without being able to see at least some large features of the pattern of that world view. In the *Meratus* example I presented above, the birth control agents needed to understand the relationship between fertility, male power, and the government.

Here is another example: In Thailand there is, to this day, a common practice of permanently curing pain by having a Buddhist monk bless a bottle of whiskey, then spray mouthfuls of the blessed liquid on the affected body parts. Understanding of this practice can be improved a little by studying Thai folk Buddhism as a belief system, understanding the role of monks in Thai village social organization, and knowing Thai beliefs about the body, health, illness, and the properties of medicines. But even with such knowledge, I doubt whether a Western biomedical practitioner would wholeheartedly prescribe the treatment, or accept it for herself. Such acceptance would require our health professional to go through a complex, orderly process of cultural accommodation, in which the Thai practice could be seen to make sense within the health professional's world view.

The process of accommodation is itself a feature of human patterning. Change, even rapid and dramatic change, is possible in two main ways: by the addition of new high-level categories in the pattern, and by the reinterpretation of existing lower level elements. Patterning has a hierarchical, or *nested* structure, like language, in which the meaning of a particular act or term is determined by the larger category of acts or terms in which it happens to participate at the moment.

As a simple example, many cultures have a context – a high-level category of behavior – we might call *teasing*. As members of such a culture, one can perceive by certain regularities in people's behavior when the category *teasing* is being performed. This perception lets us know that a special set of rules is now going to be used in the way people relate to each other. Under *normal* rules, for example, the telling of obvious lies, and the exchange of insults, would be offensive. But when the context is teasing, lies and insults are actually required, and usually enjoyable, features of interaction.

Let us return to the issue of *meaning* discussed in Chapter Three. The hierarchical structure of context and meaning can be illustrated easily in the way language works. A particular word changes meanings according to the speech context in which it occurs. If I hear only the sound *see* by itself, I do not know whether it means *see*, *sea*, or the letter "C," much less whether *see* is being used in the sense of *apprehend visually*, or *apprehend intellectually*, or *have a romantic relationship with*, or *meet with*, as in a business discussion. But the topic of conversation (higher order context) in which the sound occurs tells me which option applies. I am hardly ever confused when I hear the sound *see*, because I nearly always hear it as part of a sentence that makes sense to me.

This relationship between context, meaning, and change results in some very surprising things about human behavior, things that are hard to explain without taking context changes into account. For example, certain common actions or ways of thinking customarily used by a culture appear mutually contradictory, but people do not notice this, because they belong to different contexts. Many people in Western cultures accept the teachings of scientific physics and biology, and at the same time believe in the contradictory medieval teachings of astrology. Science is the mind set they use in their jobs, and perhaps in teaching their children, and astrology is a set of beliefs they use to understand certain mysterious things about their friends and family – such as why two people seem to be attracted to each other, or why people whom they like have certain irrational character traits.

This is how people can quickly adopt a new health practice that seems to contradict an existing one, if they perceive that the new one is effective for their purposes. The adoption may require the construction of a new high-level category of thinking, or it might require the reinterpretation of the new behavior, or the old contradictory one, or both. People who believe in the healing power of shamans to cure a particular disease can quickly learn to use modern pharmaceuticals to treat the same disease. They can decide that: (a) the same power that the shaman has (for example, to exorcise evil spirits) is incorporated in the medicine itself (reinterpretation of new behavior); (b) the shaman's rituals have the same physical effect on the patient's body as the drugs (reinterpretation of old behavior); or (c) that shamans are effective in some situations, while drugs are effective in others (new high-level distinction).

One result of this inherent adaptability of cultural patterns is that when new ideas or behavioral habits are added to the cultural repertoire, the contradictory older ones are seldom discarded – they are just relegated to a separate category. An analogy can be made to adding software programs to a computer. The tasks you can perform depend on which program is open. Patterns are flexible, but their flexibility itself follows rules. Again, an analogy can be made to language. It is easy to add new ideas, words, even dialects or special codes to a language, but it is very difficult to change either the basic grammar or the phonemics – the patterned sound system on which speech is built.

It is essential to understand the nature of cultural patterning and process in order to understand health at the community level. If a cultural way of life is subjected to rapid and massive externally imposed changes, its coherence begins to break down, and the result is a widespread moral confusion, with accompanying anxiety and depression. As we will see in later discussion of basic needs, moral order is a basic need, and its absence a potent source of physical as well as mental suffering.

As with the idea of needs, the idea of a patterned context, subject to an orderly adaptation process, dramatically affects the way CHP is conceptualized and applied. Every CHP action – indeed, every tiny detail of any action – has to occupy a place in the structured context of people's life, and the addition of any detail has to follow rules of process that are part of the structure. Some way of engaging the context and process is necessary. If this engagement is missing, several things might happen. The innovation might be ignored or rejected, it might be reinterpreted in unforeseen ways, or it might cause anxiety and conflict, as individuals struggle over how to interpret it.

However, this is not the sole, or even the strongest reason for adding the idea of patterned context to CHP. The strongest reason is that the kinds of communities where CHP is likely to be applied are those that are currently traumatized by historical change that has happened too fast. Change that occurs too fast for people to absorb in their ways of understanding and behavior results in confusion, suffering, and self-destructive ways of life. In the less-developed countries, vast and rapid restructuring of a people's way of life, a process usually called *modernization*, is being imposed from the outside, without regard to the ability of the local community to absorb the changes. In Chapter Ten, we will look more closely at the impact of rapid change on community health. Here, we can make the idea a bit more clear by returning to the concept of needs.

THE BASIC HUMAN NEEDS

Any experienced health professional knows that people regularly act in ways that increase their chances of getting sick, even when they know that they are taking this risk. Likewise, people will often refuse to take simple steps that would lead to health improvement or lowered risk of illness, even when they understand the results. Alcohol, tobacco, and drug abuse, unprotected sex, unhealthy eating, deliberate noncompliance with treatment, and dangerous sports are all common behaviors that we have tried to control by education, without much success. If we think of people as active agents in the construction of their own lives, as I have proposed, we must conclude that health is not always the highest human priority, but competes with other priorities that are often equally or more powerful. Here I propose a model of basic human needs in an effort to clarify the process by which people make health decisions.

The five basic human needs are *security, love, respect, meaning, and stimulation*. The first four of these needs have been recognized by leading philosophers and psychologists for at least 2,500 years. They are found in the work of Plato, the medieval mystics, St. Bernard of Clairveaux, Dante Alighieri, and more recently psychologists Erik Erikson and Abraham Maslow, among others (Kiefer, 1988). The fifth need, *stimulation*, comes from my own study of human evolution and psychophysiology (Kiefer, 2000). I will describe each need, and illustrate its relevance to health and health behavior.

Security refers to the feeling that nothing devastating will happen to you in a material sense – that you can count on having what you need to survive, and be free of threats to your physical being. In order to meet the need for security, you must be able to foresee an adequate income, or at least food, shelter, and the other basic necessities. You must feel relatively safe from threats of crime, injury, disease and death. A culture's economic and justice systems are critical to the satisfaction of the need for security.

Love refers to the sense of being valued by others, not because of your social persona, but for your unique self, as a person who cannot be duplicated or replaced. To be loved means to be accepted as you understand yourself to be, not as society requires you to be. It is akin to security, because such acceptance is not based on performance or capacity. Every culture creates expectations about who deserves to be loved, how, and under what circumstances. If you lack a culturally-approved loving situation – for example, if you are isolated from family and friends – you will try to establish such a situation. If a person is in a situation where he or she feels that love is deserved (for example, by being married to a loved partner, or having living parents, children, or intimate friends), but does not experience being loved, the person feels acute deprivation (Kiefer, 2000).

Respect refers to the feeling that you are valued by others as a member of society, that your abilities, status, and accomplishments are given credit. Being respected is conveyed in everyday social life by forms of speech and demeanor, and by the conferring of favors, gifts, honors, titles, offices, and employment. To lack respect means to be a *failure* and, as with love, people will risk a great deal in the search for situations and associates that grant them respect (Bourgois, 1995).

Meaning is the feeling that life is not arbitrary, senseless, or unfair, but follows rules that you can understand and accept. Much of the patterned regularity of cultural life, including religious and cosmological systems, art, literature, drama, legend, and ritual, exist largely to fulfill the need for meaning. People invest meaning in their customary surroundings and activities, and the transformation or loss of those surroundings or activities results in anxiety and depression, much like the loss of love (Frankl, 1959).

Stimulation is a need that arises from the extreme sensitivity and complexity of the human brain and nervous system. Like other big-brained animals – dogs, seals, dolphins, whales, and apes – much of human behavior is learned, and in order to learn, we must have constant input from our environment. Our way of surviving, tested over millions of years of evolution, requires us to be curious, interested, active, exploratory, questioning, and observant. We experience a lack of variety and change as a source of acute suffering. Just think of solitary confinement in prison. Culture also provides endless forms of stimulation in the form of the arts, sports, and entertainment.

To a large extent, it is the hunger for stimulation that drives our overproductive industrial economy, constantly turning out means of *having fun* that quickly grow stale and have to be replaced. In more primitive societies, small variations in the environment, the cycles of ritual, seasonal changes in diet, and life-cycle changes in relationships play bigger parts as sources of stimulation.

NEEDS AND HEALTH

Can we also say that there is a basic need for health? I believe it makes more sense to say that in addition to being a security need in itself, health is a *means* for getting the five basic needs met. What people need is a set of capacities that contribute to the satisfaction of the basic needs. In order to achieve security, a person needs the physical and mental capacity to work, to solve problems and plan, to keep his or her body and its surroundings in order. Meeting needs for love usually requires the ability to participate actively in relationships, to give as well as take. Physical, emotional, and intellectual attractiveness to others can also be important. The quest for respect requires the ability to fill respected roles in society, which in turn usually requires physical and mental competence. A meaningful life is difficult to attain unless one is psychologically able to recognize values of justice, truth, and beauty, and physically able to take action on behalf of these values. The variety and quality of stimulation available clearly depends to a large extent on one's physical and mental abilities as well – where one can go, what one can do, and how well one's senses are functioning.

Most cultures attach rich meaning to the feelings and activities shared by people in approved types of relationships, such as marriage or friend-ship. A well-matched dyad or group often agree on what is important or trivial, just or unjust, beautiful or ugly. They can help each other interpret the reality of life and make sense of it. I once did some research in Japan, comparing people who cared for a demented elder at home, with those whose parents were institutionalized. I found dramatically higher mea-sures of life satisfaction among those who were burdened with the care of the demented parent. Apparently, the meaning and status attained from this role more than offset the stress and strain. Relationships themselves provide meaning, even when one party has lost most of their ability to reflect.

In the *Coalfields* example I gave earlier, a sense of belonging to the community served people's needs for security, love, respect, and meaning. People demonstrated this sense of belonging partly by opposing outside authority – an action that reinforced their sense of respect and meaning. In the *Meratus* example, the men's opposition to the idea of birth control was based mainly on their need for respect, security, and meaning. They used the situation to compete for social status, they wanted children to contribute to their security, and they derived meaning from the Meratus model of fatherhood and leadership.

Many elderly people lose sensory acuity and mobility at the same time that the world around them is rapidly changing. As a result, they lose the ability to do familiar things and to experience a familiar envi-ronment. This is why it is so important for the frail elderly to remain in their customary environment, and to be helped to experience things *as they once were*. Sharing conversation, food, sex, sports, and entertain-ment – even quarreling – can provide a steady source of stimulation as well. These are all reasons why older people frequently become depressed when a spouse or a close friend dies.

SYNERGY, CONFLICT, AND SUBSTITUTION AMONG NEEDS

In the next section, we will discuss the process of applying the *five needs model* to the understanding of health related behavior. But first, let us look at three other characteristics of the model:

- *Synergy:* Few behaviors serve only one need; in fact, most of our complex activities are serving several needs at once;
- *Conflict:* Needs often conflict with one another, for example, an action that might improve my security, might also undermine my respected status, or vice versa;
- *Substitution:* Deprivation of the means to satisfy some needs can result in a greater emphasis on the satisfaction of other needs.

Synergy

Most of the time, people are not conscious of the particular needs that a choice or an action is meant to fulfill. One reason for this is that any given life is made up of strategies that fulfill several needs at the same time, with the same action. Consider a good marriage or friendship. A couple or small group who cooperate economically and help each other in times of need are much more secure than they might be alone. Their relationship obviously satisfies needs for love as well. The status of being married or having friends contributes to each one's respect by the wider society, as does the help each contributes to the other's career and reputation. Having others around offers many opportunities for pleasant stimulation as well.

Conflict

However, there are also many situations in life where the basic needs are in conflict with one another. My need for security and respect might suggest that I should spend the day working to earn a living, while at the same time, my need for love and stimulation might suggest that I should visit family and friends instead. I might be able to make a lot of money and satisfy my needs for food, shelter, and respect, but if the work I must do is meaningless, I will be unhappy all the same.

The basic needs can conflict with maintaining good health as well. This is particularly important for health workers and researchers to understand. Let us look at some examples of conflict between needs and health.

As I just mentioned, important personal relationships typically fulfill several basic needs. Patients will often neglect their own health needs when they perceive that these interfere even slightly with a relationship. How often have you met patients who fail to show up for an appointment because a loved one needed them at the last minute, or refuse to change a habit because that habit was shared with a loved one?

Regarding security, people will often refuse to use resources for health care if they fear they may need those resources for other things at some later time. Or, they will live with unhealthy conditions rather than move or change those conditions if they feel a general sense of security where they are. I once failed to persuade the residents of a Honduran slum to build latrines or dig gutters in their muddy streets; because they were squatting illegally on the land they feared it would be taken away from them if they improved it. They had a point.

Relatively low-status patients are often quite sensitive about the respect they get from health providers. I have talked to many patients who stopped going to a clinic or seeing a provider, or following orders, or even consulting doctors in general, sometimes with alarming consequences, because they did not feel respected in the patient role. In other words, people will give up the security of pursuing health goals in order to satisfy needs for respect.

Returning again to the story I told about heart disease in the Coalfields area of Australia, we see that it is a wonderful example of conflict between meaning and the security of health. Remember the public health authorities, worried about high rates of heart disease in the community, tried to enlist the residents in a program of exercise, diet, and education. They failed, but the residents themselves, once alerted to the problem, developed their own response: They set up a community hotline and transportation system so that people with symptoms of cardiac arrest could get to the hospital quickly. Their system saved a few lives, but why did they reject the professional intervention?

Recall that the residents viewed outside authority with suspicion and hostility, and took great pride in their ability to get along with a minimum of outside help. Evidently, they saw the cost to their meaning system of cooperating with the authorities as greater than the cost of lives if they did not. Their solution, by contrast, actually strengthened their meaning system.

Substitution

A person whose job is insecure, or who lacks access to health care, might compensate for the lack of security by putting extra energy into the satisfaction of needs for love, status, meaning, or stimulation. A person who is lonely might become more concerned with issues of respect. The example of the *Coalfields* might also illustrate this principle. This community has long been deprived of the feelings of security that derive from a good income, safe jobs, and adequate services like health care and housing. It may well be that the importance of self-respect and independence in their moral economy is in part a substitution for these unmet needs.

It is important for health scientists to understand substitution. Apparently risky or even self-destructive behaviors may often be a signal of a distorted need–satisfaction strategy, resulting from the systematic frustration of basic needs. In Chapter Ten, I explore how frustration of the need for meaning leads to a pattern of social relationships I call *self-wounding communities*.

NEEDS AND COMMUNITY HEALTH RESEARCH

Let us now apply the combined insights of *needs* and *patterned context* to community health research. In doing health anthropology, how can this theory help? I would like to suggest three ways of applying the theory. First, understanding the role of health behaviors in the local pattern of life; second, understanding the role of social change in health; and finally, understanding the impact of planned changes on health.

Assessing Health in the Context of Needs

Practical anthropological research on health generally begins by trying to understand what health problems are common in a particular community, and what causes these health problems. The second question can often be divided into health influences that are environmental, economic, genetic, and cultural or behavioral; in other words, determining the physical and economic conditions, genetic traits, cultural beliefs and practices, and individual behaviors that account for the health conditions one sees.

The *theory of needs* can be used to help understand these issues in several ways. Some questions that the theory suggests are the following:

- Given any particular influence on health – that is, environmental, economic, or cultural/behavioral factors – *how is this factor related to the satisfaction of whose basic needs?* Suppose we observe, for example, that many poor people are donating money to a local temple instead of buying nutritious food or medicine. We would ask, "What needs does this pattern of donation serve, for whom?" Or suppose we notice that local women feed their children too many sweets, with the result that the children's teeth are bad, and they are not well nourished. Who is satisfying what needs with this pattern?
- Given any particular influence on health, *of what wider contexts is this factor an integral part?* Suppose, for example, that some members of the community consult a traditional healer when they are sick, and avoid the local government health post. How might this behavior be an expression of a complex relationship between (a) beliefs and feelings about tradition, (b) beliefs and feelings about the government, and (c) the search for meaning and respect?

- Given a particular common health problem, *what is the impact of this health problem itself on the satisfaction of whose needs?* Suppose we find that hypertension is common among older people, leading to unnecessary deaths and disabilities. What is the impact of these health facts on the needs of the elderly themselves, and of other people in the village? Don't forget that some people might be satisfying needs as a result of this health problem – achieving respect and meaning by taking care of a disabled elderly relative, for example.

The Role of Social Change in Health

It is never enough to look at the health situation in a community as if things had always been as they are. All communities change, and changes affect the way people get their needs met. In most societies today, social change is very rapid. Even when such change is *positive*, in the sense that people have more wealth or more security on average, it can create a serious problem for health.

For example, rapid social change radically distorts the adaptive patterns that have been slowly built up by cultural groups for over many decades or centuries – habits that have led to the satisfaction of the basic needs. This distortion severely interferes with people's satisfaction of basic needs in communities, especially the need for meaning. The result is widespread and often acute suffering, a syndrome that lowers morale, undercuts healthy behavior, and impairs health in many ways.

Using the theory of needs in the context of social change, then, suggests the following kinds of questions:

- What have been the most dramatic local changes in technology, economics, ways of life, interpersonal relations, and beliefs in this community?
- How have these changes disrupted older patterns of adaptation and need satisfaction?
- What new strategies of need satisfaction have developed as a result of these changes?
- What are the effects of all these changes on the satisfaction of basic needs, especially needs for meaning?
- How can we understand specific health-related behaviors as responses to recent social change?

The Impact of Planned Changes on Health

Knowing something about the relationship between current conditions and behaviors on one hand, and health on the other, is extremely helpful when exploring changes in conditions and behaviors. Obviously, one does not want to make changes that would leave basic needs unmet, even while improving health conditions, unless changes are also made to meet these needs. For example, suppose you want to add prenatal and obstetric services to a local clinic in a village where traditional midwives have been handling pregnancies and births. You would want to study the midwifery service from the viewpoint of needs, and see how well you could match its functions in the new clinic. Perhaps the local women feel respected by the midwife, but not by the staff of the health post or polyclinic. They might refuse to use the new service, or they might use it but develop a bad relationship with the health service as a result.

Also, if you want to change a particular behavior – for example, smoking – you obviously want to know what needs that behavior serves, and try to think of ways to help people get those needs met in other ways. Do young people earn respect from their peers if they smoke? Or do older people find pleasant stimulation in social settings where others smoke, and expect them to do so also? How can these needs be met in other ways? Using the theory of needs, then, the researcher may ask the following questions:

- What impact will a particular proposed change have on nonhealth needs? What needs might it frustrate? How can it be made compatible with existing strategies?
- What cultural contexts will be affected by a particular change? Will introducing family planning upset the power structure in families, for example? In order to know, one must understand the symbolic meanings and power implications of sex and fertility.
- Given the need to change a behavior, what are its implications for need satisfaction? What substitutes can be found for the adaptive value of the behavior?

A METHOD FOR ASSESSING NEED SATISFACTION STRATEGIES

The theory of needs proposes that individual lifestyles and decision processes can be understood as strategies for meeting personal needs within the context of a culture and an environment. These personal strategies can be roughly understood by applying the theory of needs analytically to ordinary ethnographic data. This is a matter of studying the contents of observations and interviews while holding in mind the kinds of questions I have just listed. However, to get a more thorough and complete idea of needs and satisfactions for individuals, and to compare settings or measure change over time, it is helpful to have a standard scoring system for assessing how well or how poorly need satisfaction strategies seem to be working. The Appendix in the back of this book offers such a scoring system. Researchers who wish to use the theory of needs to understand health related behavior are encouraged to do so, adapting it to their own particular research problems and settings. The Appendix also makes the theory more concrete, by listing examples I have found in my own research of common satisfactions and challenges for each of the five needs.

SUMMARY

The existing models that are used to understand health behavior in communities and individuals generally assume that every sane adult puts a high value on being physically and mentally healthy, and if they have the knowledge and ability to choose between a healthy behavior and an unhealthy one, they will nearly always prefer the former. This chapter offers another way of looking at health behavior – that health is sometimes an end in itself, but more often it is a means to the satisfaction of other needs, needs for security, love, respect, meaning, and stimulation. These needs interact with one another in complex ways. The ways people satisfy them is patterned by their culture and environment; and changes in culture and environment disrupt need satisfaction and thereby have health consequences.

This theory of needs offers both an explanation of why sane adults often deliberately make unhealthy choices, and reveals how community health interventions often have unintended, even harmful, results. The theory allows the health researcher to: (a) search for the rational explanations behind apparently unhealthy behaviors, thereby suggesting ways to substitute healthier behaviors without disrupting the satisfaction of needs; and, (b) anticipate the effects on need satisfaction of community health interventions, thereby suggesting intervention strategies that will minimally disrupt need satisfaction habits, both for the individual and for the community.

CHAPTER TEN

Community Change: The Theory of Hope

GUIDE TO THIS CHAPTER

In this chapter we offer a model of the process by which communities are able to change common behaviors and attitudes that interfere with good health. According to this model, unhealthy communities are often those in which rapid social and economic change has distorted local culture and deprived people of a set of clear standards for working together and solving problems. In such communities, many people become absorbed in their own lives, and are not able to think about their relationship to others in a helpful way.

In order to improve the overall health of such communities, their members must develop new ways of thinking. Shared rules and ideas that support cooperation and lead to a process of group problem solving must be developed. The model offered here outlines a style of leadership that helps people to develop this new way of thinking and share it with their neighbors. The result of such a process is a community in which many people are aware of the common health problems, and are able to work together in an effort to solve them.

Throughout this book, we have been thinking about how to understand health as one outcome of a particular way of life – as the result of people trying to meet their needs according to the conditions and traditions of their community. We have argued that health anthropology is a way of understanding particular local situations, and that it is a necessary kind of knowledge for helping people to improve their health.

The great usefulness of this point of view lies in the fact that any local way of life is usually very resistant to change, even if that way of life is producing serious health problems, and even if the community's health could be dramatically improved with a few *minor* changes. Most small communities are suspicious of outsiders, with good reason. Throughout history, outside powers have sought to impose on such communities ideas that may not fit well with their ways of thinking and solving problems. Of course, communities can be changed from the outside, either by persuasion or by the exercise of overwhelming power. But unless the changes are adapted to people's own understanding of things and of themselves, the changes will not work well or last long. The most effective changes are those that people feel they are making for themselves.

If the goal of health anthropology is to help people achieve changes in their lives that improve their health, I believe the theory offered here, the *theory of hope*, can be an important part of the knowledge base of the health anthropologist. It suggests how to use improved knowledge about the contexts of health in order to facilitate change. In the next chapter, *Action Anthropology*, we will explore in detail the work of facilitating change. Here, I want to focus on how the theory of hope informs the work of health related anthropological research.

ANOMIE AND HOPELESSNESS

I have now spent fifteen years studying health and health care in low-income neighborhoods and villages, both directly and through the literature of social science and journalism. This study has informed my work with social activists in urban Honduras, Nicaragua, and California, and in rural Thailand, South Africa, Ecuador, and the Philippines – work I think of as *action anthropology*. By action anthropology, I mean the application of anthropological methods and understandings to the achievement of social and political changes – changes that are sought collectively by members of communities that accept the anthropologist as an ally.

My experience affirms the well-known fact that poverty leads directly to illness through many paths. It also shows me that some of these paths (lack of services; poor housing, sanitation and nutrition; polluted air; inferior schools; violence; public indifference) have been well studied, but there is at least one that has not: the path of lost hope.

What do I mean by the path of lost hope as a path toward illness? One of the functions of a community is to make sure everyone has what they need to survive; but it would be a mistake to think that this means only food, shelter, basic health care, and other material needs. In a modern society, it is relatively easy to provide these things, but people need much more to survive. They need meaning and hope.

To be human is to suffer. There is pain, there is death, and there are moments of meaninglessness in every life. Hope alone allows us to transcend this suffering and participate productively in the world. Without hope, people lose their humanity. When that happens, they usually need community to give their hope back, or they will become destructive to themselves and others.

Hope and meaning are closely related. The sense that life is basically just, or understandable, allows us to visualize a future in which our suffering will be explained, if not relieved. The simple act of understanding suffering in the context of a comprehensible order of things often greatly relieves it. Even the ability to have suffering acknowledged by others – that is, to make it political in addition to personal – adds meaning to it, and assuages it (Ramphele, 1997).

For this reason, most human beings are able to work, to help each other, to maintain close relationships, and find moments of contentment even in the midst of long and severe suffering. Healthy people are like bamboo – they can bend low in the worst storms of life, without breaking. History is rife with examples of humans weathering incredible challenges to mind, body, and spirit:

- During the Nazi persecutions, thousands of European Jews endured years of indescribable hardship without losing hope; most who survived went on to deal successfully with the trauma of those years, and achieve decent lives.
- In the 1940s, 110,000 Japanese Americans were stripped of their land and possessions and herded into crowded, shabby prison camps, without knowing what the government intended to do with them. Yet in their years in the camps they built thriving communities, and when they were released after the end of World War II, most achieved successful lives in the country that had imprisoned them.
- South African leader Nelson Mandela spent 28 years in prison under extremely harsh conditions, helping the entire time to lead his people to freedom, and emerging in 1990 to eventually become the leader of a new racially-integrated government.

I believe the powerful resiliency of the human spirit results from a psychological trait all people share; namely, the ability to visualize a better future, and to believe they can achieve it. This is the psychological skill we call *hope*. Hope alone allows us to transcend this suffering and participate productively in the world. The greatest heroes of history are not those who have succeeded easily, but those who have shown this awe-inspiring trait.

However, there are situations where many people within a human community seem to lose hope. These communities can often be recognized by a sense of anger, mistrust, and shame that is widely shared, and expressed in the inability of neighbors to work effectively together to make the life of the community pleasing and safe. When people lose hope, they seem to lose important skills we think of as basic for collective well-being – the ability to endure hardship patiently and work skillfully for the improvement of their own lives, and those of their families and neighbors.

When this happens to a community, the people need a process to give them back their hope, or they will become destructive to themselves and others. Once it reaches a certain level of pervasiveness, hopelessness leads unavoidably to a vicious circle of social breakdown and further hopelessness – a self-generating pathological process that destroys communities. The resulting mutual isolation, insult, and outright physical threat that members of such communities face is, in my view, one of the most serious forms of human illness.

The literature on social deviance offers a lot of theories to explain this kind of community pathology. Within this literature, several of Emile Durkheim's works, especially *The Rules of Sociological Method*, written in 1893, and *Suicide*, written in 1897 (Durkheim 1950, 1951), have stimulated a century of discussion about the effects of social breakdown on the well-being of individuals and communities. He saw this relationship as one in which accepted social norms either become unattainable or cease to make sense, as a result of social change – conditions that led him to adopt the famous term, *anomie*. Durkheim himself never systematically defined *anomie*. He repeatedly used various phrases, such as *perpetual discontent, malaise, disenchantment*, and *uselessness* to describe it. De Grazia (1949) summarizes this work, saying that Durkheim *gave anomie* three basic components: "a painful uneasiness or anxiety, a feeling of separation from the group or of isolation from group standards, [and] a feeling of pointlessness or that no certain goals exist" (De Grazia, 1949, p. 5).

Social relations in a self-wounding community show two kinds of common distortions not seen nearly as often in healthy communities. The first has to do with the substitution of need satisfactions I discussed in the last chapter. The second has to do with the widespread loss of meaning – a loss that results in a shift from positive emotions (calmness, warmth toward others, high self-esteem, optimism) to negative ones (anxiety, anger and resentment, shame).

The Substitution of Satisfactions

Even in the healthiest communities, everyone suffers from the deprivation of some of their needs some of the time, and some people suffer far more than others. But community health is supported by a cultural system, a way of life, in which most people are able to get a reasonable amount of satisfaction for a tolerable fraction of their needs, reasonably often. Families and other social networks provide people with the help they need to feel secure, the social status they need to feel respected, and the intimacy they need to feel loved.

When social rules and beliefs are clearly known and widely shared, and when there are adequate means available to live according to these rules and beliefs, much of people's need for meaning is satisfied. Levels of stimulation might be modest, but the community also shares its art, music, festivals, and conversation, and a shared set of expectations about how much stimulation is desirable.

Rapid change, especially what we think of as modernization, can disrupt this equilibrium in many ways. New technologies and sources of income require new skills and new ways of living. Economic changes force the loss old forms of social activity, threatening sources of security, respect, love, and meaning. As the values and habits of earlier generations become less useful, young people suffer confusion about what to believe and how to act. A larger number of people, especially the young, have great difficulty crafting a strategy to get their needs met, especially the first four needs (security, respect, love, and meaning), all of which depend heavily on stable human relationships and shared values.

Frustration in these four areas (security, respect, love, and meaning) often leads to the development of self-wounding behaviors as people substitute satisfactions that they are able to obtain, for those that elude them. In many cases, young people substitute stimulation for respect, security, love, and meaning, since stimulation is less dependent on stable social relations. In other cases, the loss of opportunities for love, for meaning, and for respect based on character or traditional roles, leads people to a frantic pursuit of respect by acquiring possessions and raw power. Both of these strategies tend to further destroy long-term, satisfying social relationships, as these communities become centers of aimless pleasure-seeking and vicious competition for respect, often through violent or illegal activity.

Loss of Meaning

Earlier I mentioned Emile Durkheim's works on the subject of hopelessness. Let us return to Durkheim's concept of *anomie* as a way of understanding what I am now calling hopelessness. Durkheim believed that during periods of rapid social change, communities sometimes lose their sense of certainty about what kind of behavior is good, proper, or meaningful. They lose their sense of clarity about social *norms*. Instead of working hopefully toward a more or less accepted set of goals, many people develop unhealthy feelings and behaviors. Some tend to feel depressed and aimless in a way that interferes with their work and ability to think, and might lead to isolation and self-destructive habits like drug use and fighting. Others might seek acceptance in a rebellious *counterculture*, an organized way of life that openly rejects the norms of the wider society as they see it.

As an action anthropologist (see Chapter Eleven), my definition of *hopelessness* in communities is very close to this *anomie*. Hopelessness occurs when one perceives that whatever society has promised in the way of fulfillment to its members is being withheld, through no fault of one's own, and feels powerless to do anything about it. The result is a loss of desire to seek a productive relationship with the world – a frustration and sadness often expressed in ways that are both self-destructive and bad for society.

In many American slums, for example, residents often find that the American belief in equal opportunity and self-reliance is a cruel joke. They feel excluded from most ordinary paths to success by their race, culture, language, and lack of decent education. The very institutions that exist to serve them – schools, employment offices, clinics, welfare agencies – in fact regularly humiliate them and make their lives seem meaner than ever. In many cases, the result is a sense of profound isolation and meaninglessness that seems to lead to a live-for-the-moment philosophy and a disregard for social mores in general.

Turning to the causes of *anomie*/hopelessness, one again finds Durkheim useful. He considered the cause to be a sense that the rules that one lives by, especially rules that govern one's expectations about how to satisfy needs, no longer apply. In the case of a decline in fortune or an economic disaster, the victim finds the normal expectations suddenly out of reach. In a period of rapidly expanding opportunity and wealth, even successful people likewise find the old norms meaningless, because they do not reflect actual possibilities. As I work in what I call *self-wounding* communities, I also find that hopelessness springs from a gap between expectations and realities. We live in a highly affluent society that promises equal opportunity for all, and yet systematically segregates some people in neighborhoods where extreme poverty, joblessness, poor education, dangerous physical conditions, and above all, the contempt of the wider society, are the reality.

One can ask whether a sense of unjust victimization in itself might not produce enough anger and frustration to result in the breakdown of social norms in these communities. If such is the case, there is no need to refer to the *anomie* produced by normlessness. People might simply be expressing their frustration in the only way they know how. But norms seem important when we reflect that there are in fact communities that suffer from great injustice at the hands of the wider society, and yet whose residents remain cooperative, productive, and peaceful among themselves, even apparently well-adjusted.

SELF-WOUNDING COMMUNITIES

Let us contrast conditions in wholesome, or *self-healing*, communities, with those in some I have called *self-wounding*. I draw on my own research in Honduras, Ecuador, South Africa, Thailand, and Northern California, and on the writings of Richard Couto (1991) in the rural Southern United States; Abe Kotlowitz (1991) in the Chicago housing projects; Jonathan Kozol (1995) in the South Bronx; Mark Zborowski and Elaine Herzog (1962) in the East European shtetls; Elijah Anderson (1990) in Black Philadelphia; Philippe Bourgois (1995) in East Harlem and El Salvador; and others.

Many self-wounding inner city neighborhoods have been created in the United States in the past 50 years by a kind of geographic class and racial sorting process that continues today. The most successful families move out of these areas, and less successful ones move in as the old environment becomes uglier and cheaper. Eventually, the old neighborhood contains a high concentration of racial minorities living in "problem" families: families that have only one parent or where the parents' relationship is unhappy, where the adults lack social and job skills, and where people are likely to be unemployed or underemployed, and emotionally and physically unwell.

Since the 1960s, these same communities have tended to have high rates of drug and alcohol dependency and violence. This in turn makes the better adjusted and more successful families want to move out, and leads to a steady downward trend in the community's social and economic life. Streets become unsafe, neighbors become mutually suspicious and rarely talk to each other, and a certain youth street culture develops based on toughness and risky thrill-seeking as ways of gaining social recognition. Relationships between older adults and youth especially deteriorate. This is because the norms and values that the older people understand and follow no longer make sense to the younger ones, and vice versa. Young people have a tendency to think of the older people around them as fools, and the older ones tend to be shocked and surprised by the clothing, music, language, and habits of the younger people. In this sense, you can say that there is a *culture gap* between the pre-drug and post-drug generations.

There is no doubt a close connection between the economic process and the social and cultural one. With the disappearance of well-paid low skill jobs and the deterioration of neighborhood schools, social institutions, and policing, the easy money of drug dealing and crime become increasingly attractive to young people.

Within these self-wounding communities there are always individuals and organizations that struggle to heal social relationships and give hope to those most in need. Churches, local government projects, voluntary neighborhood self- help groups, public health and welfare workers, and individual neighbors who happen to place a high value on cooperation and compassion are examples. Together, we might call them the community's *social capital*. However, as long as the forces that contribute to hopelessness and meaninglessness, taken together, continue to be more potent than the sum of efforts of social capital groups and individuals, a community will continue in a self-wounding course.

The atmosphere of hopelessness in such communities is reinforced and spread through the nature of everyday transactions between neighbors, and between individuals and institutions. A person with a low level of hope is likely to expect very little from other people, and will convey this expectation in his or her demeanor; that is, show suspiciousness and self-protection, rather than trust and curiosity. The result is usually a self-fulfilling prophecy: feeling mistrusted by others, we tend to mistrust them, and to act accordingly. It is a process that is difficult to break, for several reasons. Rowe (1999) shows, for example, that some homeless people feel justified in their mistrustful relationships with others (especially social workers), and they congratulate themselves for being "too smart to be fooled" by people who say they want to help them. In other words, they use the only power they have – the power to refuse to cooperate with any plan or accept any offer that does not meet their terms. Under the circumstances, even the most well-meaning sources of possible help in self-wounding communities often burn out or become discouraged, and either leave or stop trying to do a good job of helping people.

Under these circumstances, small cooperative groups of a dozen or two individuals tend to form, especially among young people. Such groups are based on two principles: first, shared loyalty and trust, and second, an attitude of resistance toward external control of all kinds. Kids essentially form small counter-culture cliques, devoted to opposing the adult world – the school, the law, and older people's values in general. A good deal of youth gang behavior, as well as music and entertainment culture (which is paradoxically controlled by the oppressive wider society) can be understood in this light. Elijah Anderson's study of social change in a Black Philadelphia neighborhood (Anderson, 1990) documents this. Older people, once respected as "wise heads" and effective at enforcing community norms of politeness and cooperation, are now seen by the young as having a value system and view of the world that is irrelevant. I have found the same thing in South Berkeley in recent years.

SELF-HEALING COMMUNITIES

The contrast between these conditions and those of what I call self-healing communities is useful. As I study self-healing communities I discover a process of cooperation and hope building that goes on in all of them.

They have developed a set of beliefs that they can call their own. They think about themselves in a way that is different from, and better than, the way their oppressors think about them. Sometimes this set of beliefs is based in religion, sometimes in a sense of their own history and culture. These local beliefs give meaning to the community's own special experience of life. They lead to norms of behavior that honor mutual cooperation, and draw people together in mutual respect.

This alternative might be a widely held minority belief and ritual system, like the Judaism of the East European *shtetls* (Zborowski & Herzog, 1962); or the Mayan traditions in rural Guatemala (Benitez, 1992); or it might be a local tradition of civic pride, as in some rural Black towns in the American South (Couto, 1991). Studies of these communities indicate that the mere ability of a community to thrive – to educate its young, shelter its poorest and most vulnerable, and protect its property and values against constant attacks – in the face of a hostile environment, forms the basis for meaning and cooperation. The tremendous impact of Marxism on the urban poor can be understood in this light: Marx explained the suffering of the early industrial working class in terms that made sense to many of them, and created the basis for new norms of solidarity in impoverished communities.

In self-healing communities, people tend to look at each other and themselves not as potential exploiters, but as *brothers and sisters*, people who share the common experience of oppression. Empathy and kindness tends to grow out of that experience. It is as though the shared experience itself provides the basis for the development of a local microculture, in which norms of mutual respect, protection, and kindness eventually prevail. Janey Skinner (2003) studied *peace communities* in Colombia, oppressed by drug dealers, local militias, revolutionary guerillas, and the national army, and actually documented the development of this ethos over a period of months.

Mutual help naturally grows from the expectation that people have of each other, that they will be respected and treated kindly. The result is not just an emotionally healthy social life, but a population with an average level of self-esteem and hope that is relatively high. The boundaries between these local self-healing communities and their wider society is of course a problem. The values of cooperation within the community keep hope alive, but they are usually based on distinctions between *us* (people who are members) and *them* (people outside the community's boundaries). Remember the story in Chapter Nine about the people in the Coalfields: They would cooperate with each other to improve emergency services, but they were determined not to cooperate with the outside authorities to reduce heart disease rates. We will return to this problem later, when we discuss the role of the researcher in directed community change.

THE PROCESS OF COMMUNITY EMPOWERMENT

The important question for health researchers interested in practical results is whether, and how, self-wounding communities can be transformed into self-healing ones. Here, Durkheim's theory may have useful implications. When confronted by a community of *anomie*/hopelessness, the action-oriented anthropologist seeks measures that might change the situation. One seeks to help communities develop a set of norms that can reverse the process and produce a sense of belonging and meaning, in turn reducing social pathology. Here, reports on processes of community organizing for change, often called *empowerment* or *capacity building*, seem to support Durkheim's theory.

The work of community empowerment generally begins by helping residents to better communicate with each other. The new communication process has two characteristics: (a) it focuses on shared perceptions, feelings, and needs; and (b) it does not exclude anyone, but treats everyone equally, and shows everyone respect. Using this democratic process, the community tries to reach some agreement on what kinds of things need to be changed first.

Once some kind of agreement has been reached, several new things can happen:

1. People can begin to work together to set shared goals, outline strategies, and carry out mutually beneficial work.
2. Gradually, while they are spending time working together respectfully, people get to know each other, to trust each other, and to talk about things they have in common. Each one begins to realize he or she is not so different from others, and need not mistrust them so much. As trust and friendships grow, people unconsciously begin to agree on many things – in other words, new norms start to develop – norms that are in keeping with the real lives of community members.
3. The work of achieving shared goals gives members an opportunity to experience the rewards of cooperation. As a result of this, cooperation as a norm is reinforced within the group.

4. As cooperation and a shared set of beliefs and values gradually emerge, *anomie* and hopelessness gradually shrink away. Those who participate, let's call them the activists, find themselves feeling better and enjoying life more.

5. Other members of the community, observing the work of the activists, begin to see that those who participate seem happier. Some nonparticipants begin to join the activists, to learn the new shared norms, and to spread these new norms to still others in the community. Interestingly, community activism often continues in this way for many years, even in the absence of real solutions to the problems the activists were originally trying to solve. The rewards of simply having something in common to work for are so great, that the work continues even when it never succeeds.

All this suggests that Durkheim's theory of *anomie* may be useful in several ways. First, wherever we see rapid social change, we should look for a sense of confusion and sadness, caused by a gap between people's expectations and their lived realities. Second, we should look for shared signs of illness and disharmony in such communities, signs that are caused by this alienation and hopelessness. Third, we should seek the path to healing this condition by helping to establish new norms that more closely match the local community's immediate realities.

Helping People Understand Themselves

The work of the anthropologist is of little practical use to the communities we study unless it helps those communities understand themselves in a way that leads to positive change. If we are interested in helping (and why else study community health?) we must not only satisfy our own curiosity, we must shape our findings to the information needs of the people we study. According to the *naturalistic theory of knowledge*, this is what social science is for. A good theory, then, is one that makes sense to the people it describes.

The *naturalistic theory of knowledge* holds that the test of a theory is in its usefulness, not merely in its logical power or the fineness of its agreement with the facts. We do not do research to test the absolute validity of theories. Rather we use theory as a tool, to help us construct and refine a useful intuition of a problem we want to solve. So it is with the theories offered in this book, the *theory of needs* and the *theory of hope*. To illustrate this, let me outline an alternative theory of community change, one that might end up being more useful in a particular community than the theory of hope.

An Alternative Theory of Community Change: *Street Marxism*

I believe many of the people I have worked with in low-income communities would reject the theory of hope as a description of their condition. First of all, they would say that I am making something simple seem very complex. The fact is, poor people feel powerless when they view their lives in isolation, but when they have leaders that help them confront their shared problems together, they realize they can act effectively, and they do so. They would say that no new standards of behavior are necessary; only clarity about how to organize themselves to act on what everyone already knows to be just and right – the right to participate fully in society and share its wealth with tolerable equity.

Second, they would point out that Durkheim's analysis fails to put the blame in the right place. Rather than focus on the unfair practices of the rich and powerful, it implies that poor people cause their own problems because they don't know how to act. In fact, they would say, poor people know that the institutions of the ownership class are to blame for the problems of their communities. They would say that this kind of belief about the poor is sold to the general public by the news and entertainment media, which are owned by the upper classes. They would point out that many ghetto residents act out their anger on one another, not in ignorance, but from sheer frustration and a lack of power to confront their real oppressors. Peaceful oppressed communities, they would say, simply have not suffered enough to be pushed over the edge into uncontrolled rage. As proof of this, they could point to the many cases in which people have eased their oppression not by peaceful organizing alone, but by their willingness to act violently if necessary (Katz, 1989).

Many of my friends in low-income communities would note that Durkheim's view of poor individuals is itself insulting. It implies that most poor people are slavish imitators of custom, lacking the imagination and will to make up their own goals – goals that will work for their own lives. Worse yet, they would say, the theory of hope implies that the idea of a social conscience is an illusion! It implies that community reformers are unaware of their own dependence on their social group, and suffer from the illusion that they are following universal ideals such as human equality and dignity.

Many of my working class friends would know that this street analysis owes a great deal to the Marxist tradition in social science. Whatever its origins, it makes a good deal of sense. It resonates with the personal experience of many residents of many poor communities. It suggests individual action against oppression, claiming that there are universal values beyond the norms of both the local community and the oppressor class. It offers a view of the relationship between individual and society that encourages responsibility and action, based on one's intuitive understanding of justice and human dignity. Finally, it fits with the fact that the self-interest of the wider society is often held in check by the threat of violence from below.

USING THEORY TO HELP PEOPLE CHANGE

Let us look at these two theories of community change – the *theory of hope* and the *theory of Street Marxism* – and imagine how each of them might be useful in helping communities improve their health. In keeping with our model of how knowledge is built, we will ask, how does the theory help us specify the parts of our intuition about community change? And how does the theory help us to identify cases for comparison?

The Theory of Hope

In the case of the *theory of hope*, we might begin developing the parts of our intuition about community change by asking five kinds of questions:

1. Where are the points of conflict, confusion, and despair in the local culture? Who seems to disagree with whom, about what? What strategies are people using that do not produce good results? Who often feels unhappy or confused, and about what? What prevents people from cooperating when it is clearly in everyone's advantage to do so? How is conflict and despair expressed?
2. Where are the points of hope and harmony? Who agrees about what beliefs or issues? What does everyone seem to feel proud of? What do people enjoy doing together? What tasks can they cooperate to accomplish, and how? Who is able to solve disagreements, and how?
3. Who are the opinion and work leaders in the community? Who do people turn to for help or advice? How do these people work, and what do they believe? Are they generally successful at promoting hope, or not?
4. What is the role of specific changes in technology, economy, environment, and culture in promoting or destroying hope? What has happened to work, family, community, learning, religion, leisure, and health, and with what effects on morale?
5. What efforts has the community made to improve its conditions? What have been the effects of these efforts, both on objective

conditions, and on the morale of the activists? Who joined the efforts, and why?

Turning to our second area of inquiry, the identification of cases for comparison, the *theory of hope* suggests the following issues and questions:

1. *Cases of individual confusion and despair.* About what issues do people express confusion, hopelessness, and pain? Note that the state of confusion or despair itself usually expresses a lack of clarity on the part of the sufferer about the explanation of the problem. A teenager might say, "My parents are too strict, they don't understand my needs," while the parents might say, "She wants to imitate her friends, who smoke, wear sexy clothes, and hang around with boys." The underlying issue might be a new form of marketing on TV that encourages children to buy things their parents don't want them to have.
2. *Cases of conflict between individuals and groups* – young and old, rich and poor, men and women, different religions, occupations, political groups, and community versus outsiders or authorities. What values are at stake in these conflicts? What is their effect on community life?
3. *Cases of isolation and avoidance that keep neighbors from forming ties.* What prevents people from friendly interaction?
4. *Cases of specific, concrete change in the cultural environment.* A new technology, a new kind of work, a new law, a new food, new knowledge, even a change in leadership. How do people use it? How do they talk about it? What does it do to their lives?

The Theory of Street Marxism

Let us follow the same exercise for the *street Marxist* theory of community change. This theory holds that action is possible when communities understand the unfair practices that deprive them of their rights, and have a method of organizing in order to confront and change those inequalities.

What might constitute the parts of an intuition based on these ideas?

1. The most obvious measures would be those of actual positive and negative treatment of community members by outsiders. Evidence of differences in opportunities for education, jobs, housing, health care, credit, and political office or influence. To be really useful, the data would have to be specific and concrete, showing not just differences in outcomes, but differences in access. What

specific individuals or organizations take what specific actions that have the effect of denying or granting equal rights to members of the community? One important measure of cross-boundary interaction is simply who participates (community members versus non-members) in various kinds of social, political, and economic activities in the surrounding area? An absence of community representation supports the theory.

2. One would also want to collect data about images of the community held by outsiders. By looking at the way outsiders write or talk of the community in local news and conversation, one could develop a clear picture of negative attitudes. Again, one would need to identify specific individuals, institutions, and situations that express negative stereotypes.

3. Another feature of the inequality proposed by the theory might be the results of cooperative efforts by community members (and their allies) to reduce inequalities. Under what circumstances have such efforts been successful or unsuccessful, and why? Who have been the leaders and the joiners? What styles of leadership have proved effective? What were the results in terms of community morale and overall cooperation?

Regarding the identification of cases suggested by Street Marxist theory, one would want to collect data about the following:

1. Actual interactions between community members and outsiders, either individually or in groups. To what extent does a given interaction (job application, medical encounter, request for help, etc.) reflect discrimination?

2. Local laws and practices that regulate the access of community members and others to needed resources. Are they fair nor not?

3. Incidents of political and other cooperative action that affect community well-being.

4. Individuals and groups who either support or oppose the rights of community members.

There are, of course other theories of community change, and other models of how it can be achieved. Some models emphasize the need to bring outside resources into the community or to build cooperative groups of communities who share similar problems, in order to have major influence on the remote sources of power that affect local conditions. Although I have said that all social truth is local and time limited, I see no reason why anthropologists cannot be involved in projects of directed change that reach beyond the communities they study. And I actively recommend that any and all theories should be explored in the search for the most useful research intuition.

SUMMARY

Health anthropology often serves the goal of helping people change behavior or the environment, or both, at the community level. Experience has shown that this is hard to do, but the *theory of hope* offers a model of how successful communities solve shared problems. The theory holds that in troubled communities, rapid social change has undermined the shared expectations and standards of meaning and behavior that are necessary for people to trust one another, believe in the future, and cooperate for the common good. The process of community empowerment can, under certain conditions, begin to heal this loss of trust and hope. It is a process in which a small group of activists, with strong leadership, establish new norms of community cooperation, and gradually propagate these norms among their neighbors.

The theory of hope suggests that the health anthropologist should look specifically for processes that result in the increased exchange of helping behavior and information, in decreased mistrust and mutual harm, and in more expressions of hope and trust among community members.

The theory of hope is contrasted with another model of community change, *Street Marxism*, in which the mechanism of change is thought to be increased control by community residents over the resources (jobs and income, infrastructure, housing, education, public services, civic decision making) that affect their well-being. In stressed urban American communities, street Marxism is often the model most familiar and persuasive to the residents themselves.

CHAPTER ELEVEN

Action Anthropology

GUIDE TO THIS CHAPTER

This chapter explains a special type of research called *action anthropology*. In this type of study, the role of the researcher is not just to observe and analyze life in a community, but also to participate in a partnership with change agents in the community in order to help them achieve goals that they select for themselves.

Action anthropology is very different from the type of academic research most of us have been trained to do, because it requires the researcher to accept the values of the local change agents who are partners in the work. This often involves taking a stand *against* certain points of view that oppose the changes that the partners are trying to make.

Action anthropology is completely compatible with the naturalistic theory of knowledge outlined in Chapters One through Four of this book. In doing action anthropology, the researcher acts as an equal with those studied, seeks results that are useful, and places the knowledge acquired in the hands of the community. However, to be most effective, the action anthropologist must often use leadership skills in addition to knowledge gathering and analytic skills. He or she should know something about how voluntary organizations function to get work done, and should be able to help local partners make good decisions about how to lead people and achieve change.

This chapter, then, describes the process of voluntary cooperation for social change, and explains how action anthropology can contribute to that process.

RESEARCH AS COMMUNITY PRACTICE

Health itself being a goal of human society, research on the health of communities nearly always has a practical aim, no matter what theory of knowledge it is based on. The naturalistic theory of knowledge holds that truth is largely a matter of *usefulness*. The usefulness of anthropological research is one of the main themes of this book. But the idea of usefulness is far from simple in the human world, for several reasons:

1. Usefulness means different things depending on one's perspective. A spider's web is useful to a spider, but not to a fly. A clever advertisement might be useful to the salesman, but because of it I might buy something that is useless to me.
2. A potential user of a thing might have to be taught its usefulness first. Many users who were initially skeptical of e-mail or cell phones, for example, now find them vital in their professional or personal lives.
3. Making use of one good thing often requires giving up another. I might have enough money either to buy a bicycle or to get my computer fixed, but not both. If I take time to read books, I have to give up practicing my guitar.

Being clear about different views of the usefulness of knowledge is extremely important in community health practice (CHP). CHP is based on health promotion and disease prevention, which means changing a community's usual ways of thinking and living. This requires cooperation between health experts and local residents, and cooperation in turn requires some kind of agreement about what is useful and important. Clearly, if the health researcher is to make a lasting difference in people's lives, she must not only understand their needs, but also help them see themselves in new ways that will encourage them to change some things about the way they live.

This chapter is about the process of achieving cooperation between health experts and communities. It is based on the *Theory of Needs* (Chapter Nine) and the *Theory of Hope* (Chapter Ten). Accordingly, health is viewed not only as a goal in itself, but also as a means for the satisfaction of basic needs, within the context of community life. The struggle to improve health, in other words, must promote, not diminish, people's feelings of being secure, respected, and loved, and their sense that life is meaningful and interesting. Any practical actions that result from health research must support these goals, but that is not all. The relationship between the researcher and the community itself must embody these goals as well. A researcher who interferes with people's self esteem and sense of meaning will be working against whatever health goals she is trying to promote.

The Empowerment Process

In Chapter Ten, we discussed how self-wounding communities can be healed by collective action to solve their own problems. When people in such communities unite to discuss shared problems, make plans, and take action to solve those problems, several things can happen:

1. Community members can learn that they are not alone – that there are many others in their community who feel as they do. This in itself is an empowering experience.
2. They can begin to trust each other more than before as they experience working together. Each one appreciates the support and friendship of the others.
3. They can begin to have the pleasant experience of success at planning and carrying out meaningful work. This makes them realize they are more powerful and more skillful than they thought.
4. Their values can begin to change. The well-being of the community becomes more and more important to them, and other, more selfish needs become less important.
5. Their lives can become happier, and they often become healthier, because their work together fulfills many of their needs for respect, love, meaning, and stimulation – and sometimes security as well.

This is what is meant by the term *empowerment*.

Notice that for the process of empowerment to succeed, the active members of the community must experience this process as something they do for themselves and their neighbors, not as something that they are instructed to do by outsiders. People first must reach the understanding that they need to change some things in their community for their own sake. Then they will gladly learn from others what they need to know to carry out their plans.

Most communities need some outside help in starting this process of empowerment. The kinds of help they may need are:

- organizing informal community gatherings, where people feel free to talk openly about their problems and think creatively about solutions;
- collecting information about the real health problems in their community, the causes of those problems, and some possible solutions to them;
- organizing work in group sessions where specific goals are set, people are assigned tasks and taught how to do them, and schedules are made;
- carrying out projects in the community – making sure the work gets done properly, on schedule, and that mistakes in the plan are discovered and corrected in the process;
- evaluating the effects of actions and using these evaluations to modify the plan or carry out new actions;

- sustaining the process of empowerment, by making sure morale in the group stays high, that leadership is strong, that conflicts are resolved, and that new people are continually recruited into the process.

Action Research Adds a Moral Dimension to Science

What I am calling *action anthropology* is the process whereby the researcher takes the role of outside helper in promoting the process of empowerment. It is important to notice how this role is different from the usual work of researchers.

Traditionally, social science research has occupied two different positions in society. First, there is that of *academic* or *pure research*, the quest for knowledge that is driven less by human needs, than by the leading intellectual questions that interest the community of scholars at the time. It is often spoken of as the work of advancing theory, or filling in the gaps in basic knowledge. Academic researchers are usually employed by universities or private research institutes. Examples of academic social research would be the attempt to understand the health of a certain community by applying stress theory, or an attempt to find new ways of measuring cooperation and conflict.

Second, there is *applied research*, where the scientist aims to use her knowledge and skills mainly to solve practical problems, and not so much to advance the state of science. This might sound similar to action anthropology, but again, it is different in an important way. Traditionally, the applied researcher is employed by government or industry, and her work is directed by her employers. While members of the community under study might have some voice in deciding what the research goals and methods are, they do not control these things, and the results of the research do not belong to them. Their principal role is to be the "material" that the researcher tries to transform according to goals that are set by others. An example of traditional applied research would be trying to reach national health goals for cardiac health by comparing various kinds of exercise and diet programs in a community. Another example would be to study the effectiveness of various teaching methods, in order to produce textbooks for a health education business.

Action anthropology, by contrast, begins with neither the goals of science, nor the goals of social change agents outside the community. Although the action anthropologist might be paid by a government agency, university, or private non-profit organization, her goals are set by the community under study, and the results of her work are made available to the community to use as they see fit.

This difference might sound simple, but actually it is very difficult to achieve, for several reasons. Some of these reasons we have already discussed in Chapter Six. In every society, a scientific knowledge is defined as a form of expert knowledge, something that is potentially valuable for the society, that takes a long time to learn, and that few people possess at a professional level. The successful professional scientist is by definition a high status person, and the products of his or her work are by definition high status products. The idea of poor people being able to employ a scientist, or being able to use the work of a scientist as they like is difficult for most people to understand – especially other scientists! People tend to mistrust what they do not understand.

Another difficulty faced by action anthropology is that the work it produces is a potential source of power to the community that receives it. Action anthropology often produces information that poor communities can use to challenge the practices and laws that regulate their lives and affect their health. Whereas any kind of social science research might reveal that government or commercial practices are harming a community, action anthropology produces this knowledge for the *community in question*, in a form that community members can use in their own interests. In most cases, this feature of action anthropology creates mistrust among those who already exercise power in the community.

In short, action anthropology is far more than just a technical skill. It is, in a very real way, a moral position as well. To do it takes more than a mastery of ideas and techniques. It takes courage.

THE ACTION RESEARCHER AND COMMUNITY EMPOWERMENT

Earlier I defined *empowerment* as a collective process undertaken by communities themselves to solve their own problems. This appears to be a contradiction. If empowerment is an independent local process, in what way does it need the researcher, an outside expert? There are two principle ways in which most communities need outside help to begin addressing their collective health needs: first, to assist in the development of community self-awareness, and second, to act as a liaison with the outside world.

Developing Self-Awareness in the Community

In almost every human community, there are a few people who recognize that the well-being of members could be improved if everyone would cooperate to change things. Typically, these people are either too few to begin the process of empowerment by themselves, or they lack the skills, or they cannot agree on where to begin the work, or they mistrust each other too much to discuss the matter at all. Often all of these obstacles keep things from changing. In addition, there are often many people in a typical community who would like to solve their own problems in cooperation with their neighbors, but they either: (a) do not realize that their neighbors have the same difficulties they do; or, (b) do not know what process could get people to begin cooperating. People in poor communities, especially, often have a long history of frustration over trying to change things, and develop the habit of thinking that nothing can be done.

What such communities need, in order to begin the process of empowerment, is information about what the shared problems are, and about what steps they can take to begin building cooperation. In the first stages of change, this is the kind of information that a researcher can help them realize. It is not a matter of *teaching them how to think and what to do*, however. If the researcher takes the role of teacher, the experience for the community will be disempowering – people will feel that once again, they are dependent on outsiders. Rather, as we shall see, the action anthropologist simply helps people create the conditions for self-discovery and independent action.

Creating a Liaison Between the Community and Outsiders

The need for health anthropology as a kind of study arises because the cultures and environments in which most professional health workers and government administrators live and work are very different from the cultures of the local communities they serve. The health anthropologist functions partly as an interpreter, helping residents and outsiders to understand what each other mean, how they view each other's actions, and what course of action by each group might maximize the chances of cooperation between them.

For example, when local government provides resources for a community empowerment project, they usually want to receive regular reports from project leadership, indicating exactly what has been accomplished. It is often necessary for the action anthropologist to explain to community members, in terms that fit their understanding, why such measurements are necessary, and what kinds of information would be helpful to the administrators. At the same time, it is also necessary to explain to the administrators why the kinds of measurements they would like to have (for example, number of children immunized, or quantity of education materials distributed) might not be good indicators of project progress.

Another common liaison problem has to do with professionalism and control. Health providers and bureaucrats are used to exercising control over those areas of community life in which they have expertise. But the very exercise of control might be undermining the community's sense of its own effectiveness, and damaging the process of empowerment. The

Coalfields example, quoted in Chapter Nine, is a good illustration. The residents did not want the health authorities to tell them how to live; they wanted to solve the problem of heart disease in their own way.

The Limitations of the Action Researcher

There are some unusual features of action anthropology that the researcher needs to think about before undertaking such a project. First, even more than naturalistic research itself, the empowerment process usually takes several years. The researcher should either plan on being available to the community for as long as it takes, or should have a plan to transfer his expertise to people who will be able and willing to help with the work until native leadership is ready to take over.

A related issue is that there are many unforeseeable problems that can reduce the effectiveness of the empowerment process. Conflicts can develop within the community or within the activist group. Opponents outside the community might organize to stop the work. Changes in the political, economic, or physical environment might reverse the work or make it irrelevant. These are simply things that can affect every effort at social change, but their risk for the researcher in action anthropology is magnified, because the process of empowerment requires that the activist group and the community be encouraged to experiment with their own ideas and learn from their own mistakes.

DOING ACTION ANTHROPOLOGY I:
KNOWING THE COMMUNITY

We are now ready to discuss the actual process of action anthropology in a step-by-step fashion. Of course every community and every empowerment project is different, so the guidelines given here must be adapted for each.

As mentioned in Chapter Seven, the more the action anthropologist knows about the research community, the better. In the best case, the researcher should have a thorough understanding of the local culture, history, and environment, and be able to understand a good deal about how the problems identified by the community are related to the needs, power positions, and perceptions of various stakeholders, and how they are expressions of wider cultural patterns and historical trends.

Of course, this ideal situation is often impossible in practice. Agencies that fund community development and health projects typically work on schedules that do not allow researchers enough time to learn the situation this thoroughly. Accordingly, let us try to identify the most important areas of knowledge for the action anthropologist. At the very minimum, before taking an active role in facilitating social change, the action researcher should learn as much as possible about the following issues:

1. *The structure of power and influence.* What individuals and groups are the most powerful, and the least powerful, in the community, and what are the sources of their power? Who are the *opinion leaders* – those whose ideas are the most trusted or admired – and who are thought of as offensive or ineffective, and why? How is power negotiated in the local culture?

2. *The major problems and their recent history.* What health and social problems are widely felt to be important in the community? How long have they been problems, and what do people believe has caused them? Given ongoing changes such as migration, technology, and economic and cultural trends, where do these problems seem to be heading? What are some leading opinions about what to do? Which groups hold what opinions about each problem? What collective efforts have been tried to solve these problems, with what results?

3. *Community resources.* What are the potential resources and strengths of the community for purposes of working together to solve problems? Are there trustworthy leaders? Is there goodwill between neighbors? Are there organizations that know how to direct work? Is there an effective system of information sharing? Who has special abilities, such as teaching, writing, speaking, construction, research, or organizing? Who can provide support for collective work in the form of space, food, transport, equipment, supplies, money, or special knowledge?

4. *Major stakeholders and stakes.* Who might be benefiting from the community's problems, and who is likely to be hurt by them, and how? What is the history of relations among the stakeholders, and how is this history likely to affect the dynamics of change? Such relationships need to be calculated not just within the community, but between the community and outside constituencies as well. For example, if joblessness is a problem, what are the opinions about the community of potential outside employers, and how has this situation evolved?

Benefits and harms need to be calculated not just in material terms, but in terms of needs – status, love, honor, meaning, and stimulation – as well. For example, if drunkenness is a problem, local liquor sellers probably benefit materially, while the families of heavy drinkers probably suffer most. But there are other stakeholders and other values to consider. Drinking might be part of a cultural complex that strengthens bonds among, and gives meaning to, many drinkers. Drinking might provide a cheap source of stimulation for many with dull lives. Either the promotion of drinking or opposition to it, or both, might be an important source of political power for some. Money from the sale of alcohol may play an important part in supporting community organizations such as churches and clubs. The making and transport of alcohol might be important income sources. Those who gain from alcohol-related behaviors, such as those in the fields of sports, entertainment, prostitution, and gambling, might gain from it as well.

DOING ACTION ANTHROPOLOGY II: FACILITATING CHANGE

Earlier in this chapter I discussed the *empowerment process*. There I listed the kinds of help members of a community usually need in order to start the change process. Here, let us describe in more detail how the action anthropologist can help with each step.

Organizing Gatherings and Sharing Information

Initially, there are four main purposes of community gatherings to initiate the empowerment process:

- so that people can express their own concerns to their neighbors and leaders, and feel that others are listening to them sympathetically;
- so that they can hear that others in the community feel the same kinds of things they feel – they are not alone;
- so that they can experience the feelings of respect, hope, and trust that occur when people demonstrate interest in each other, and in their community; and,
- so that those most interested in helping to change the community can identify themselves to each other for future planning.

The success of these initial meetings is critical. In the average person's everyday life in modern society, they often feel completely unimportant and helpless. They are used to being told what to do by so-called experts, and being ignored if they disagree or try to contribute to collective life. Since it is painful to experience other people's indifference, the ordinary person usually gives up complaining or trying to change things, and does not realize that others share their problems. *Initial community meetings should provide as many people as possible with the feeling that there are others in the community who care about their problems and respect their ideas.* This nurtures people's need for respect and meaning, and provides the first small feelings of empowerment.

The initial meetings provide the organizers with an opportunity to demonstrate giving respect to everyone present. This is a key attitude and skill that will continue throughout the process. If those who attend have a chance to feel respected, they will be much more likely to attend future meetings.

The strategy for organizing such meetings will need to differ according to the local culture and history. One must make sure that people are not afraid to say what they think – they must feel that there will be no bad consequences of expressing themselves openly. This refers to feelings as well as material consequences. The least powerful segments of the community especially must be helped to feel secure. One key to success is to make sure that the organizers of the initial meetings are individuals who are well known and widely trusted by those who attend.

It is important that the opinions and feelings expressed at initial meetings actually represent a broad range of community opinion. One common mistake made by organizers is to allow the most outspoken people to dominate. The opinions of such people might not reflect the community as a whole, and the individuals themselves might be widely disliked and mistrusted.

It is important to keep good records of what is said in the initial meetings, and to have a system for sharing this information, not just among those present, but throughout the community. This information forms the basis for future meetings. The action anthropologist should do her best to keep records of what opinions are most popular, how opinions may differ between different social groupings, what possible sources of cooperation and conflict can be identified from the discussion, and what individuals might have the skills, social characteristics, and interest to help lead the empowerment process.

Organizing Work, Collecting Facts, Evaluating Actions

Some communities already have people who are well trusted and liked by ordinary people, and who have the skills and time to organize empowerment work, and others do not. The key organizers must have three sets of skills. First, they must know how to analyze complex problems into clear, simple tasks, and lead people in accomplishing these tasks. Second, they must be able to help people build confidence in themselves. Ordinary people develop confidence by discovering their own abilities and knowledge, making decisions, accomplishing goals, and enjoying respect and admiration for their work. Third, they must be able to encourage mutual trust and affection among the active participants, and between the active ones and the rest of the community.

The goals of accomplishing work and building self-confidence are difficult to balance. Often, work gets done more quickly and with fewer problems when it is organized and directed by a strong leader. However, simply following orders does little to increase self-confidence. For that, it is best if leadership and decision making are spread widely throughout the group. This in turn often means that the group must spend much more time discussing decisions, and might also mean that the members of the group might have to learn their skills by making and correcting many more mistakes.

The leaders of an empowerment process must be able to steer a course between these two principles. This is a skill that I cannot teach in this chapter. The correct formula will differ according to the culture of the community, the personalities of the work group, and the nature of the problems with which they are dealing. The most important message here is that accomplishing community goals through an empowering process takes a long time.

The *Look, Think, Act* Model

One of the great benefits of the community empowerment process is that a rich knowledge of the problems it addresses is already present in the group that will undertake the work. People who live in the community usually know who is involved in causing a problem, who suffers the results, and some of the solutions that have been tried and failed. They may know many of the stakes and stakeholders, both for the problem itself and for any planned solution. They may know where some of the resources that are needed to change the situation can be obtained.

However, this local knowledge is usually not clear and focused. Pieces of it are scattered among community members, who need to work together to put those pieces together. Exactly as with naturalistic research, once the work of clarifying the problem begins, the community will discover that certain needed pieces of knowledge are missing, and they may need help in searching for those pieces.

EXAMPLE: A Self-Help Group Learns to Connect People with Jobs

The Community Outlook Improvement League (COIL), was a group of neighbors, residing in a low-income city area called "The Flats," who had joined together to improve local health. Early in their work, they recognized that unemployment was responsible for many local health problems. People who could not find jobs were more likely to be involved in crime and drug abuse, less likely to be well-nourished and housed, and were also poor role models for younger people.

When the COIL members studied the employment problem, they found that there were many low-skilled jobs that local people could do in the nearby suburbs. They began to publicize these jobs in local barbershops and hair salons, but no one took them. When they interviewed jobless people in the community, they found that it was difficult for local people to take these jobs because few of them owned cars, and the public transportation system did not connect the community and the job-rich areas.

The members of COIL and their friends now had considerable useful knowledge. They knew: (a) where many of the desirable jobs were; (b) many of the people who needed these jobs and could do them if they had transportation; (c) where the job seekers lived; (d) what hours these people would need to travel to get to the jobs; and, (e) where and when the existing public transport routes ran. They tried writing letters to the bus company complaining about the lack of transport, but this had no effect. A low-level transport company manager wrote to them and explained that it would be too expensive to change the bus schedules.

When they discussed the situation further, they identified some things they did not know about the problem, such as: (a) what the process was for reviewing transport routes and advocating for change; (b) what the costs would be to the public transit company of the changes they wanted; and, (c) how to organize community members and local elected officials to pressure the authorities for the changes.

With a little help from their leadership, COIL members learned that if they had this information they might be able to improve the situation. They then organized themselves and got the information through telephone calls and meetings with local officials. And finally, through trial and error, they managed to get about twenty members of the neighborhood involved in going to public meetings and speaking to the press about the problem. In the process they learned a good deal about how local government works, and how to organize people to take action on a shared problem. They also got the attention of several local officials and community members, who were now more willing to listen to them. Eventually, they did get some new bus routes added, and this success made them very proud and happy, and improved their image in the neighborhood.

The members of COIL had used the basic strategy of community action, called the *look, think, act* model. First, they looked at health problems in the community, and discovered that joblessness was a factor in many of them. Second, they thought about the problem of joblessness and formulated an action plan that might help. Next, they looked at the results of their action, and saw that it did not work. Looking further, they learned more about the problem, thought about this new knowledge, and designed another action. When this too failed, they looked again at the result, thought what more they could do, learned some new facts, and took still further action.

Some things to notice about this process are that:

- it allows people to learn by practical experience, which is probably the most efficient and thorough way to learn skills;
- it works through cooperation and promotes teamwork;
- it simplifies complex problems into small concrete steps, so that people starting out with modest skill levels can gradually build confidence and ability; and,
- it encourages patience, thinking, observation, data collection skills, and perseverance, things that people can use in many other settings.

Sustaining the Process

In order for people to continue to put energy into a project, their work must continuously meet some of their basic needs. They must feel personally admired and appreciated by others whom they care about, satisfying needs for respect and love. They must continue to believe that the work of the group is important and that they are making progress, satisfying needs for meaning. The work must be varied enough that it holds their interest, satisfying needs for stimulation. Their needs for security must also be met, and the work must not threaten their sense of safety and optimism. In short, sustaining the empowerment process depends on the ability of the most active participants to develop a culture among the participants that: (1) sustains the satisfaction of most participants' needs, most of the time; and, (2) continuously draws new people into the process, either as active participants or as passive supporters.

The role of the action anthropologist and other leaders of the empowerment process is to model and teach the cultural attitudes and skills that sustain satisfaction. The best description of the needed attitudes and skills I have seen is the work of Ernest Stringer, in his book, *Action Research* (Stringer, 1996). Stringer divides his cultural principles into four areas: relationships, communication, participation, and inclusion. I have modified a few of his items in order to make them fit better in non-Western cultures.

Relationships in action anthropology should:

- promote feelings of being respected and liked for all people involved;
- maintain harmony;
- avoid conflicts where possible;
- resolve conflicts when they arise, openly and with equal respect to everyone;

- accept people as they are, not as others think they ought to be;
- encourage personal, cooperative relationships, rather than impersonal, competitive, conflicting, or authoritarian relationships; and,
- be sensitive to people's feelings.

In effective *communication*, one:

- listens attentively to people;
- accepts and trusts what they say;
- can be understood by everyone;
- is truthful and sincere at all times;
- acts in socially and culturally appropriate ways; and
- regularly shares information and advises others what is happening.

Participation is most effective when it:

- enables everyone to be actively involved;
- encourages activities that participants are able to accomplish for themselves;
- enables people to perform meaningful and significant work;
- provides support and encouragement to people as they learn to act for themselves; and,
- deals personally with people, rather than with their representatives or agents.

Inclusion in action anthropology involves:

- maximizing the involvement of all relevant individuals, that is, anyone who has an interest in the process and wants to participate;
- inclusion of all groups affected;
- inclusion of all relevant issues – social, economic, cultural, and political – rather than focusing on narrower administrative or political agenda;
- ensuring cooperation with other groups, agencies, and organizations; and,
- ensuring that all relevant groups benefit as much as possible from activities.

This list of rules makes it seem rather simple to develop a culture of empowerment, but of course this is an illusion. In practice, it is very difficult. Every individual human being is unique. Each person sees the world differently, and has slightly different needs in any given situation. The job of creating harmony and cooperation can be extremely complicated. The proper role of the action anthropologist in the empowerment process is to combine the *perspective of the researcher*, which we have been discussing throughout this book, with the *perspective of the activist*, someone who is committed to the improvement of community life through cooperative action.

The *researcher* takes the roles of:

- a student, always curious about and respectful of what people think and how things work, only giving an opinion when asked;
- a participant, learning while doing as local people do;
- an analyst, looking for regularities and explanations in the complexity of everyday life; and
- a communicator, helping people both within the community and beyond it to achieve useful insights into local life.

The *activist* takes the roles of:

- an ally and participant, willing to take on assignments (including leadership if necessary) decided by the group in order to advance the collective cause, contributing on a daily basis to the solution of problems and the completion of tasks;
- an advisor, ready to offer the perspective of an expert if asked;
- a role model, helping others develop the cultural skills needed by using those skills within the group and demonstrating their results; and
- an advocate, explaining the needs of the group to outsiders, and supporting their requests for support.

Perhaps the most important skill for an action anthropologist, however, is *adaptability*. The process of empowerment is always long, complex, and unpredictable. There are always unforeseen problems and new challenges. The action researcher must always be alert to changes in the dynamics of the activist group, in the progress of the work, and in the larger political and economic climate, and must be able to change tactics to meet the evolving situation. This should be a familiar idea by now, as it is a necessary part of the naturalistic method of research we have been discussing throughout this book.

SUMMARY

Action anthropology is clearly useful as a way of forming partnerships between health scientists and members of the communities they study and serve. I believe this method also has an important intellectual function, however. The naturalistic theory of knowledge and its philosophic origin, pragmatism, hold that usefulness is the ultimate test of truth (see Preface). Action anthropology provides a powerful way of putting our knowledge to the test of usefulness. If we, as scientists, can help the people we study to develop solutions to their own problems, I believe we can say, in a way, that we have *proven* the *truth* of our ideas.

Of course, this has been a goal of social science since its beginnings, over a hundred years ago. As I mentioned at the beginning of this book, the results have not been very encouraging. Why should we believe that action anthropology represents an improvement on traditional methods in this respect? I believe the answer is this:

Because of the complex, open-ended nature of society, social change is never complete; it is an endless process, whose results are never certain. When the members of social communities themselves are active in the process of solving their collective problems, they themselves learn ways of seeing and acting that allow them to observe the results of their actions, and continue the process of searching for better solutions. Through action anthropology, communities not only learn these skills, they also develop the necessary optimism and self-confidence to use them.

CHAPTER TWELVE

Teaching Health Anthropology

GUIDE TO THIS CHAPTER

In this chapter I describe the methods my associates and I use, which I call *student-centered teaching* and *problem-based learning* – methods of social science instruction that are more appropriate for naturalistic anthropology (and in my view more effective in general) than the traditional teacher-centered method widely in use.

For 18 years, my associates and I have been teaching 50 or 60 health science students each year in my anthropology classes. During and after each one of these classes, some of the students come to us to thank us for the experience. They tell us things such as, "This class changed my life," and "This is the best class I have ever had at the university." Often, we see these students later on in their careers, and they usually like to remember the classes we had together. I see this as a positive comment on the effectiveness of our teaching approach.

TEACHING AND RESEARCH SHOULD GO TOGETHER

As we have seen, the relationship between the researcher and the community under study in naturalistic anthropology is quite different from that of positivist research. Under the naturalistic method, the researcher aims to join and blend in with the community, in order to establish trusting relationships and see things from the local point of view as much as possible. This method is incompatible with the role of the researcher as an *outside expert*, one who seeks to speak directly to other professionals, rather than to the ordinary people whose lives provide the substance of her expertise.

Naturalistic research usually requires that the researcher spend long periods working independently in field settings. The study setting is likely to be very unfamiliar to the researcher in the beginning, and the work requires self-confidence, patience, and a playful attitude toward one's work.

Also, there are likely to be many situations where choices must be made between equally attractive explanations of complex findings, or equally intriguing directions of further inquiry. The researcher must have a high tolerance for uncertainty and ambiguity, and must be able to make difficult decisions with confidence.

There are powerful similarities between the naturalistic approach to research and a nontraditional approach to teaching.

Traditional Teaching Methods

Traditional methods of teaching social science have been better suited to the positivist approach than to the naturalistic one. By *traditional methods*, I mean the widely-used model of academic classes, in which the teacher takes the parent-like role of final authority, disciplinarian, and example for the students. In this model, the students are required to absorb new knowledge and practice new skills, and it is always the teacher who decides what should be learned, how, and at what rate. The students exercise choice, if at all, mainly in deciding which courses to take. In many institutions, even that decision is dictated by the student's advisor.

Each individual student submits his or her performance to, and receives knowledge and grades from, the teacher. The most important relationships are then between the teacher and each individual student. Among each other, students compete for approval, especially if the teacher grades *on the curve*, assigning failing grades to the worst performances.

Under the traditional system, students learn that there is a right way and many wrong ways to do the work. This approach is useful in fields like mathematics, languages, and some aspects of physical science, where the objective is to eliminate ambiguity in the results. However, it has severe limitations in the social sciences in general, and it is disastrous for learning the naturalistic theory of knowledge. As we discussed in earlier chapters, naturalistic research does not seek to identify any absolute truth, rather, it seeks to produce a subjective view of life that is maximally useful. There might be many useful views, depending on the needs and thinking habits of the audience.

A Better Way: Student-Centered Teaching

What is needed for the teaching of health anthropology as we have presented it, then, is a method that does several things differently. The proper method should:

- present a model of the scientist (that is, the teacher/facilitator) not as an expert authority, but as a skillful student, full of curiosity and creativity, eager to learn from others, accepting of ambiguity, and unafraid of making mistakes;

- create a social atmosphere not of competitiveness but of mutual respect, trust, and interest among the students – an atmosphere as close as possible to that which the researcher strives to create in the research setting;
- create an atmosphere in which the students are not inhibited by the fear of being wrong, but willing to test the persuasiveness of creative ideas in a safe situation where they can count on honest but respectful discussion;
- generate a diversity of ideas, so that students can compare solutions to problems and assess their relative usefulness and persuasive power;
- support student self-reliance, confidence, and enthusiasm for the lengthy and sometimes uncertain tasks of independent data collection and analysis; and
- convey the lesson that knowledge and learning are open-ended; that there is always more to know, and that this is a good thing, not a sign of failure.

The student-centered teaching method aims to achieve these goals by the application of the following eight principles:

1. Classroom activity that is based on open discussion and exchange among all participants, not on lecturing or teacher-dominated exchange.
2. Careful attention at all times to the emotional atmosphere of the learning group, in order to create a climate that stimulates openness, creativity, and confidence.
3. Using the teacher/facilitator role to model curiosity, respectfulness, and flexibility, rather than authority and control. This includes reduced social distance between the teacher/facilitator and students, and between the students themselves, in order to build learner trust and confidence.
4. Focusing on the learning process rather than on the "correctness" of answers, in order to encourage diversity, experimentation, and tolerance for uncertainty.
5. Maximizing student responsibility and teamwork in the learning process, in order to develop autonomy and decision making skills.
6. Using students' interests as a major basis for selecting learning material.
7. Frequent use of complex actual situations as learning experiences, in order to develop students' ability to confront the complexity

and ambiguity of real human social systems, and to help them develop the social skills needed for naturalistic field work.

8. Using *problem-based learning*, which we will discuss in detail below, as a way of understanding the process of research in a concrete, personal way.

Benefits and Costs of the Student-Centered Method

I have been developing and using the student-centered method for eighteen years. I believe it is not only better suited to naturalistic anthropology, but that it is also more effective as a way to teach social science in general, and perhaps other subjects as well. In my experience, students enjoy this method because:

- it helps to fulfill their needs for respect and gives them plenty of pleasant social and intellectual stimulation;
- when students are enjoying themselves, they are more relaxed and able to think creatively;
- giving more responsibility and respect increases their motivation to work, as does encouraging students to pick problems that are most interesting to them personally; and,
- having them solve problems in real situations increases their ability to remember what they have learned, and to apply it effectively in their own work.

Also, you will notice a close similarity between the student-centered method and the method of community empowerment discussed in the last chapter. These two processes work, I believe, basically the same way. As people begin to experience working in a close group based on trust and respect, four important things happen. First, they begin to trust and respect themselves more, so they are able to work more effectively. Second, as they discover their own abilities and receive respect for them, they become more motivated to do the work. Third, this positive shared experience makes them more willing and more able to cooperate with others. Fourth, having learned these things, they are better able to lead and teach others, both within the learning group and beyond it.

The *main cost* of the method – and it can be a very serious cost – is that it requires close interaction between the teacher/facilitator and each of the students. Accordingly, it is easiest to do in small groups; it loses its effectiveness among larger classes. It also requires more teacher/facilitator time to prepare and administer than most traditional classes. Student-centered teaching is high quality teaching, but like most high quality things, it tends to be costly.

THE METHOD OF STUDENT-CENTERED TEACHING

Here I will discuss the basics of class size, selection of students, location, resources, scheduling, and preparation.

Class Size

The ideal class size for student centered teaching is between six and fifteen. Since interaction between students with a variety of different viewpoints is important, fewer than six may not be satisfactory. While it is possible to work with classes larger than fifteen, it becomes more and more difficult as class size increases. This is because it is important for every student to be able to participate actively in the class, and to be able to feel that his or her participation makes a difference. Later, we will discuss some ways of improving student participation in larger classes.

Selection of Students

If possible, it is best to bring together in the classroom students who have different ideas and personal life experience, but who have about the same level of preparation. To some extent, the class sets the pace and level of learning. If some students are much more advanced than others, either the more advanced ones may become bored and frustrated as the less prepared ones struggle with basic material, or the less prepared ones will become discouraged and stop trying to keep up. It works well to mix men and women, older students and younger, and even students with different educational goals, such as medicine, social science, and nursing. If all the students have a strong interest in using health anthropology in their careers, this of course is best.

Location

As with any other class, it is best to have a well-lit, cheerful room where people feel comfortable. I like rooms with large windows that let in natural light and air, but often this is impossible. The room should not be much bigger or smaller than is necessary for people to be comfortable. A good-sized room helps create a feeling of closeness in the group. (However, it is not the most important thing. I have held successful student-centered classes in some very strange places – including out-of-doors and in vacant biology laboratories.) It is best if the chairs or desks in the room can be arranged in a single circle, or around a single table, so that everyone can see everyone else's face, and so that people feel equally included and respected. The teacher/facilitator should sit in the circle or at the table and at the same level with everyone else.

Classroom Resources

It is important to have a means to display the class's activities of the day – and sometimes of earlier days as well – where everyone can see them. This can be done by using blackboards, poster pads, an overhead projector, or a laptop computer connected to a projector. The means of display should allow for changes to be made easily, to reflect frequent changes in the class's thinking. If classes are long, or held during students' usual meal times, it is useful either to provide food or to allow students to bring their own.

Scheduling

Student-centered classes can be scheduled either as intensive *immersion* courses, in which students spend their entire study time with a single class for several weeks, or as one of several classes in a diverse curriculum, meeting a few hours a week. I recommend that student-centered classes be scheduled for at least two hours at each meeting if possible, for two reasons. First, the interactive seminar nature of the class requires that students get to know each other and the teacher/facilitator reasonably well. Longer class sessions help this. Second, student-centered classes are more enjoyable and more instructive when the students are able to discuss complex issues in depth. Often, classes start with rather superficial questions, but move toward more complex and difficult ones as the discussion proceeds. Less than two hours is usually too short for these sorts of deep discussions. I also recommend that classes should meet at least once each week for at least eight weeks. Longer breaks between classes may cause the emotion that builds up in the seminars to dissipate, lowering the quality of the experience. Shorter course durations also make it difficult for the students to get to know each other well enough to build up sufficient trust.

Preparation

The usual preparations for class include careful explanation to the students of the goals and content of the course, the methods used, the assignments and expectations of the students' performance within and outside the classroom, principles of grading, and basic student conduct during discussions. In addition, it is important for the teacher/facilitator to explain the *principles of respectful discussion* and *student responsibility* that the class will be expected to follow. Explain to the students that the success of the class depends on their active participation. This in turn means that every student, without exception, brings useful skills, experience, and viewpoints to the class, and that the goal of the class is for everyone to learn from, as well as teach, everyone else.

In order to achieve this, it is necessary that each student:

- does all the assignments and attends all the sessions;
- comes to class prepared to discuss the assignment for that session – that is, to ask and answer questions, take positions, add information, or make observations;
- actively respects every other student, by listening carefully to their comments without interrupting, taking turns when speaking, limiting their own comments to the topic under discussion, and being mindful of other students' feelings throughout the term of the class; and,
- thinks critically and speaks openly, not only about the content of the class but about its overall structure and process as well – that is, if a student thinks more or less time should be spent on a particular topic, or that other learning materials or methods would improve the class, she should say so.

ROLE OF THE TEACHER/FACILITATOR

Seiji Ozawa, the great symphonic conductor, once said, "Conducting an orchestra is like pulling on a heavy weight with a rubber band. If you don't pull hard enough, you get no movement. If you pull too hard, the band breaks." Student-centered teaching is a little like conducting an orchestra. The skillful teacher/facilitator seeks a balance between leading and simply supporting the students. The main tasks of the teacher/facilitator are the following:

1. To design the learning plan and select the content that will be covered in the class – up to a point. Giving the students permission to add to, or change, the content so that it better meets their needs and is in keeping with the principle of giving responsibility and respect.
2. To explain the learning process and the dynamics of the class to the students. Students must understand what is expected of them, and why.

3. To model the behavior of a scholar and teacher/facilitator in the naturalistic tradition. The teacher/facilitator:

   • shows an eagerness to learn from the class and from each individual student, demonstrating how naturalistic research and teaching is done;

   • shows respect for every student, listening actively, praising useful contributions, remembering details that are important to students, helping them when they have difficulty both in and between classes, giving responsibility whenever it is appropriate, deferring to the students whenever they might be able to take initiative in learning.

4. To maintain an emotional climate in the classroom that promotes learning, that is, one that is relaxed, curious, playful, enthusiastic, energetic, and confident.

5. To evaluate the progress of each student and of the class as a whole continuously, to see where the learning experience is succeeding and where it needs to be improved.

6. To revise and adjust the learning plan and content continuously in order to improve the effectiveness of the course.

Classroom Strategies for Creating Student Confidence

As I mentioned above, classroom activities in student-centered teaching are designed to involve the students actively in the learning process, and to model the idea of naturalistic knowledge as the search for useful solutions to problems, rather than the positivist idea of *correct* answers to empirical questions.

Given these rules, the student-centered method pays close attention to the emotional climate of the learning experience. There are two reasons for this. First, learning takes place more rapidly, and knowledge is remembered better, when students feel relaxed, curious, and confident. It is the job of the teacher/facilitator to create an environment that supports these feelings. Second, the work of the naturalistic social science researcher in the field will be more successful if he or she is able to sustain these same emotions, and to inspire them in others, throughout the research work. Every teacher/facilitator is free to experiment with strategies for creating this emotional climate in the classroom, but here are some methods that I and other teacher/facilitators have found useful.

Humor

Every human situation that is not completely tragic contains possibilities for humor. Without getting away from the serious topics that the class is studying, the teacher/facilitator can make use of the humorous possibilities of these topics, and encourage the students to do so also, as long as they are careful not to embarrass each other.

Learning Games

There are many short, interesting games students can play that ease tension and keep energy levels high. For example, at the start of class, I sometimes ask each student in turn to say their name, and then the name of a fruit that starts with the same letter. Each student in the sequence must say the names and fruits of all those who went before him, before saying his own. This helps students learn each other's names, which contributes to the social success of the class. Sometimes I have several students stand close together and play the game *human knot*. In this game, each person randomly takes the left hand of another person in their right hand, and takes someone else's right hand in their left. What results is a tangle of hands, arms, and bodies. The students are then told to untangle the knot, without letting go of hands, and without taking both feet off the floor. It can always be done, and it always makes people laugh. This game builds self-confidence and teamwork. There are books that list many such games.

Brainstorming

There are many forms of the *brainstorm*, the exercise in which the teacher/facilitator (or one of the students) simply asks the class to give as many answers as they can think of to a question, while someone writes all the answers on the blackboard or poster sheet. The class can then do several things with this list: (a) they can explain why each item answers the question; (b) they can group the answers into categories according to their similarities and differences or (c) they can try to apply these same answers to a different problem. And so on. From this, students learn critical thinking, and they have the advantage of having their view of a problem broadened, by seeing everyone else's answers. This also gives the teacher/facilitator an excellent opportunity to build student confidence, by praising the answers, and allowing students to show their reasoning skills in a safe environment.

Debate

When students are studying an intellectual problem, the teacher/facilitator can get the class to list several possible solutions to the problem. Students can then be assigned to teams, each team required to develop the arguments in favor of one particular position, and present their arguments to the class. This exercise: (a) forces students to be creative, especially if they do not like the position they have to defend; (b) usually generates humor, when students think of outrageous defenses for their argument, or when they playfully insult the arguments of other groups; and (c) builds teamwork, as each team must work together to build their strategy. To add pleasure to the game, the class as a whole can vote for the team they feel won the debate.

Role Playing

When students are required to learn a skill, such as analyzing a social system, the class can be divided up into groups who take different roles. Suppose you are using the example of a village where the teenagers are abusing alcohol as an analytic problem. You can have one group of students pretend to be teenagers, another group be parents, another be the police, and a fourth group be health workers. Then each group can try to explain the situation from the viewpoint of those roles. If you are teaching interview skills, you can divide the students into pairs, one of which will be the interviewer, the other the subject, and then reverse their roles.

Team Problem Solving

Classes can be divided up into small teams, of anywhere from two to six members. The number in each team needs to be small, so that each student in each team can play an important role. Each team is then given a problem to solve together either during class or as homework, which they will present to the class. This of course creates teamwork and mutual trust, and it also gives an element of competition to the class that strengthens motivation. It improves learning, because the whole class can see the different strategies that teams used to arrive at their solutions.

Active Participation

Active participation of all students is important. It is during participation that the most rapid learning takes place, and the teacher/facilitator also needs to observe each student's performance in order to evaluate and adjust the teaching. Depending on the size of the class, and the differences between the learning levels and personalities of the students, it is common that some students are more active than others. A danger in giving the class responsibility is that some students may come to dominate the class, while others become less and less active. The teacher/facilitator needs to observe this, and make sure everyone is as active as possible during class discussions. This can be done in several ways: by asking direct questions to students who tend to be silent, rather than waiting for them to speak, and likewise, asking students who have already had a turn to speak to wait until others have had a turn.

Or, the teacher can follow a *check in* procedure, in which each student in the room is asked to speak in turn. Less active students may be assigned projects, which they then report on in class. Or, the instructor may have students take turns leading the class, as described later.

Films, Videos, and Guest Speakers

As with any other class, having the students watch short segments of film or video in class can be an excellent stimulus for discussion. Material should be emotionally vivid and cover more or less the same themes as the readings. This is especially true of guest speakers. In teaching about a particular social problem, I find that the students particularly benefit from hearing speakers who are not professional teachers, but who have had extensive experience as ordinary citizens or as clinicians with the kind of problem we are discussing. For example, in my course on poverty and health, I often bring in social workers or nurses and their low-income clients. Students can often learn far more from such people's experience than they can from an abstract analysis of the problem. In these sessions, I make sure that the speaker and the students can exchange ideas.

Student Facilitators

An excellent way to motivate students to learn the material well, while building their confidence and modeling the learner role of the scholar, is to arrange for the students themselves to take turns co-leading the class. In many of my classes, I assign groups of students (usually two or three) to work together to devise a plan for leading a given class. I help them prepare their plan, but during the actual class, I have the students ask the questions and direct the discussion, while I, as teacher/facilitator, interfere only when I feel it is necessary. This also helps to make the class lively, as the other students are exposed to different methods of teaching from mine.

Food

This might sound strange, but I find that student-centered classes are more successful if simple food and drinks are provided at every class meeting. Eating and drinking have several positive effects on learning. They increase blood sugar, making people more alert and energetic. They make people feel secure and cared for, which lowers tension levels and makes social interaction easier. They also help to create an atmosphere of friendship, in which students' good feelings about each other (and the teacher/facilitator!) are easily expressed. At times, I have had the students take turns bringing snacks for each other; at other times, I have provided the food myself. In the latter case, some students always bring a few things also, just to show their appreciation and their liking for the other students.

Classroom Strategies for Larger Classes

Sometimes it is not possible to hold classes with small groups of students. However, some student-centered teaching methods can also be used in large classes of 30 to 100 or more students. Here are some ways this can be done.

Ask Questions of the Class

The instructor can ask questions of the students in a large class, either waiting for some students to volunteer the answers, or selecting some students by name and asking them to respond. Of course this must done in a spirit of exploration, curiosity, and fun, and not be threatening or intimidating to the students. There are several methods to accomplish this goal, such as the following:

1. Start with easy questions, or ones the students are interested in and know something about. For example, ask them to talk about their own experience with something familiar to many of them, such as "how it feels to be sick," or "what happened when you had to lead a group," and so on.
2. Explain that you yourself do not have a good answer to the question, but you want to learn from them what they think about it.
3. At first, point out to the class only the good points about whatever answers you receive. Don't contradict the students in front of the group. If you get a really good answer, repeat it, and say why it was good.
4. Use humor. Make the dialogue between instructor and students amusing.
5. Prepare the students in advance. Tell them before the class meets what kinds of questions you will be asking.

Have Groups of Students Take Turns Preparing Presentations

Tell the students ahead of time that they will need to get together in groups to prepare presentations to the whole class. Have a plan for how to form the groups, then meet with each group outside of class to help them plan a good presentation. Presentations can be short or long. One way to do this is to pass around a sign-up sheet with the class topics listed on it, and ask for people to sign up for the topic they like. You can shift people around if there are too many or too few for a given topic. At the end of the students' presentation, point out what was good about it, then ask the entire class to comment constructively on it.

Have the Class Form Discussion Groups

Even a large class can spend time in discussion among the students. Help the class arrange itself in groups of six or seven to discuss a particular question or problem, within a limited time (usually half an hour or less). Each group should have a *reporter*, who will report to the class as a whole, briefly, the results of the group's discussion.

These methods encourage the students to study the material, build their self-confidence, and help them to feel proud of their learning. More importantly, having the students take responsibility for teaching reduces the power distance between instructor and student, and models to some extent the ideal relationship between researcher and community in naturalistic research.

Group Teaching

Some social science courses are taught by a group of faculty, rather than a single teacher. Because student-centered teaching is based on close interaction between the students and the teachers, it is important that the members of the teaching group are able to communicate with each other closely. Every teacher must understand and agree closely on the goals of the course, the methods to be used and the purpose, the faculty's expectations of the students, and how to handle common problems such as poor student performance or disruptive attitudes or habits. Inconsistency among faculty styles or expectations will be bad for both the students and the teachers. This does not mean, of course, that faculty members should try to teach exactly alike – *the personality of each teacher is valuable* in itself, and the students can and should learn to accept slight differences in style.

The teaching group should therefore meet regularly to discuss these issues, or at least should communicate often by e-mail. I mentioned earlier that student-centered teaching works particularly well if there are two instructor/facilitators present at each class meeting. One way to assure consistency of teaching methods throughout a faculty group is to have each faculty member paired with each other faculty member for at least one teaching session.

HOMEWORK AND OUTSIDE ASSIGNMENTS

As with in-class exercises, there are a variety of outside assignments that can be used to introduce students to anthropological inquiry.

Reading Assignments

Since the heart of student-centered teaching is in class discussions, it is important that every student should come to each class well-prepared. Being prepared means that everyone has read the same material and thought about it carefully. Careful thought means *questioning* the viewpoints expressed in the reading, and *applying* the material to one's own experience and one's own needs and interests. Occasionally, I assign audiotapes, videotapes, or even movies in the theaters as well as readings.

For each class session, the students should learn two or three important ideas that can serve as the basis for discussion. I believe the quality of the students' thought about the reading material is more important than the quantity of what they read, so I recommend relatively short reading assignments.

Journals

When I first began student-centered teaching, I learned that I needed direct one-on-one contact with each student outside of class, so that I could listen to their ideas and concerns, and learn how each one's mind worked. This knowledge helped me shape the class discussions and homework assignments so that they addressed the students' needs. This was a bit complicated, because it meant the students and I had to arrange meeting times and places outside of class.

After a few years, however, one of my assistants, Kira Foster, suggested that it would be simpler and more efficient if we asked the students to keep personal journals of their thoughts about the class, and turn these journals in to us regularly. This turned out to be a wonderful idea. Now I always have my students informally write down their ideas about the class each week, and either give the written journals to me in person, or e-mail them to me. Each week I read all these journals, and make comments on all of them. This greatly strengthens and enriches the dialogue between student and teacher/facilitator. This way, I can attend specifically to each student's concerns, encourage their good ideas, and raise questions that they need to think about. The topics of these journals range widely, covering everything from their recommendations of things I have not read, to brilliant original analyses of the material, to statements about their own anxieties concerning the class and their careers. Reading all the journals is time consuming, but I think it is time well spent.

Field Work

There is a saying teachers use: "If you hear it, you forget it. If you see it, you remember it. If you do it, you know it." Collecting and analyzing anthropological material are skills that cannot be learned from classroom study alone. Students must observe actual communities, do real interviews, and struggle to understand what they have found. They need to put personal experience together with learned concepts. In this way they will come to *know* the steps described in this book. Knowing something means understanding how it functions and why it is important, not just because you trust the source of information, but because you have had the personal experience of having used it to your own benefit, in your own life. This is a form of *problem-based learning*, the next topic of this chapter.

There are so many ways of doing field work, so many kinds of problems that students can choose, and so many kinds of settings where they can study them, that I will not try to give examples. Rather, the following are some skills that might form the *learning objectives* of field work assignments.

Seeing Similarities and Differences

All human communities are highly patterned. In some ways, all communities are alike (for example, people have to have shelter and food, raise children, and settle disputes). In some ways culture, environment, and history create distinct regional patterns (for example, the types of housing, the way food is grown and prepared, what children are taught, and how arguments are settled). And in some ways every community is unique (the exact arrangement of houses and the history of each one; who prefers one kind of food or another; which children were raised this way or that; and who fights with whom about what). Yet in our everyday lives, we are usually not conscious of these patterns in human environments and behaviors. One of the first tasks of doing anthropology is to learn how to see them, and begin to understand how they express local life.

One of the exercises we do with some of our classes is to take them to two different neighborhoods in San Francisco – an upper-income one and a lower-income one. We ask them just to look at the houses, streets, shops, people, cars, and parks, and tell us what patterns they see, and what they think these things mean. Are there metal bars on windows? What kinds of things are sold here? How are the people dressed, and how do they behave? What kinds of pets do people have? In one low-income district, there are many small parks in the middle of crowded streets, with children playing there. There are also many brightly painted murals on the walls of buildings. What do such things mean? The research process typically begins with questions such as these, which lead the researcher gradually deeper and deeper into the history and culture of the community.

Taking Notes

Students have to learn the basics of note taking. What sorts of things need to be recorded? How does one take notes without disturbing people? How can one record things quickly, so that little time is lost? What kinds of recording apparatus are the most effective?

Participant Observation

Students might be asked to do some volunteer work in the community, as part of a research assignment. This way they learn such things as how to explain their role to local people, what culture shock and being an inept outsider feels like, and how to use participation as a way to build rapport and get information.

Interviewing

Interviewing practice helps students learn how to approach people about volunteering, how to schedule interviews, how to establish rapport, protect people's privacy, encourage open conversation, ask questions in the language of the interviewee, take notes while talking, and manage their own feelings about difficult topics or difficult respondents.

Analyzing Data

Actually taking notes and analyzing them teaches such important skills as: What kinds of questions or observations yield the most useful information? How does one record information so that it can be found most easily later? What steps in data management seem to work best?

PROBLEM-BASED LEARNING

There are now many books on *problem-based learning* (PBL) as a way of teaching complex skills efficiently and effectively. The basic principle of PBL is that students learn faster and remember better when information is learned in the process of solving a real (or realistic) practical problem. (Note how well this complements the naturalistic theory of knowledge – that *truth* equals *usefulness*.) Another important advantage of PBL is that it helps students *learn how to learn*, that is, it requires them to be active learners, to essentially teach themselves and each other the knowledge and skills they need to solve the problem. In this way, it allows them to experience personally some of the qualities of a mature scholar: self-directed problem solving, use of professional materials and techniques, and so on.

In simplified form, the steps of PBL are:

1. A group of students (usually three to ten) is given a complex prob- lem that requires for its solution the kind of knowledge they are learning. If it is a class in medicine, the problem might be a patient with a particular set of symptoms, a particular history, age, gender, and so on; the students' job being to diagnose the patient's illness or injury. If it is a class in anthropology, the problem might be a social or health problem in a particular community, with a certain culture, environment, and history. The students might be asked to make some recommendations to the public health department about how to begin addressing the problem.

2. The students are asked to discuss the case among themselves, and to make hypotheses about what might be causing the problem, based on their knowledge of the science and of the case. Using the naturalistic theory, we would call this the formation of an intuition of the problem. If the problem is well chosen, the intuition will contain several plausible hypotheses, and these are written down. The teacher/facilitator might ask them questions about why they made a particular hypothesis, in order to stimulate clearer think- ing, but should not interfere in their decisions at this point.

3. The students are then asked to discuss this list of hypotheses, and make a list of other things they need to know in order to eval- uate each one of the hypotheses further. In naturalistic theory, this is called *specification* of the parts of the intuition. The miss- ing knowledge might be a list of observations of facts about the case that will rule some hypotheses out, or it might be technical knowledge about what sorts of things are theoretically linked to the problem. Usually it is both.

4. The students then divide up the work of getting the knowledge needed to improve the list of hypotheses, either by narrowing it down, or by finding new hypotheses that might fit better. Each student might take one or several questions, or a small group of students might take a particularly complex question and subdivide it. This work is typically done as homework, since students must spend time seeking the knowledge needed. Knowledge collection might include studying other cases with similar findings, which in naturalistic theory would be called *comparison of cases.*
5. Once this new round of knowledge has been gathered, the students meet again to reconsider the original intuition, or list of hypotheses, and refine it. Depending on the time available for work on the problem, steps 3 through 5 might be repeated, or the students might offer their best hypothesis at this time.
6. When the class in question has an applied or action focus, the students then make a list of recommendations about how to relieve the problem.
7. The teacher/facilitator and the students review the case together, and discuss what problems came up during the exercise and how they solved them, as well as ways in which the analysis and the solution might have been done better.

EXAMPLE: A Problem-based Learning Exercise

Our goal was to teach anthropological data collection and analysis methods to a group of eight Thai nursing faculty in our student-centered course in San Francisco. We felt it would be easiest for our students to have a problem where they could use a familiar language. Because there is a sizeable Lao community in San Francisco, Dr. Jeremiah Mock, my associate, arranged for the students to interview several elderly Lao who use a multicultural senior center in the city.

Step One, Choosing a Problem: We began by discussing with the students what they would like to learn about the elderly Lao. They chose the problem: "What are the main challenges and resources for health of the elderly Lao in San Francisco?"

Step Two, Building an Intuition: The students then thought about the question, and came up with a list of hypotheses about what they thought the main challenges and resources would be. The list looked something like this:

Challenges: 1. lack of money; 2. lack of access to basic services; 3. inability to speak English 4. lack of knowledge about health care, nutrition, and exercise; 5. dangerous environment (too much crime); 6. poor housing; 7. social isolation and loneliness due to lack of opportunities to meet other Lao, or to travel back to Laos for visits with family and friends.

Resources: 1. Strong families; 2. other Lao in the area; 3. government health insurance; 4. knowledge of traditional medicine.

Step Three, Designing an Interview: The students then made a list of the questions they would need to ask the elderly Lao in order to refine their intuition.

The list included questions about: 1. each person's age, occupation, when they came to the United States, where they currently live, and who is in their immediate family; 2. health problems and feelings about their health; 3. their income; 4. how often they see a doctor, where they go for medical services, and what they think about the services there; 5. whether they have health insurance; 6. what languages they speak, and how well; 7. whether they have non-Lao friends; 8. what they eat; 9. how they exercise; 10. whether they feel safe where they live; 11. what their housing is like; 12. where their families live; 13. whether their families help them; 14. how often they see other Lao, and where; 15. whether they are lonely; 16. whether they have been back to Laos or not, whether they plan to go, and how they feel about that; 17. whether they know or use traditional Lao medicine.

Some time was spent designing each question so that the elderly would be sure to know what was meant by it.

Step Four, Doing the Interviews: The students divided into teams of two, and each pair interviewed at least two elderly Lao for about an hour, on two separate occasions if possible.

Step Five, Analysis: After the first interviews, the students compiled the results. They found that: 1. very few elderly worried about money, and although many had little, they felt their standard of living was adequate, compared with what they had in Laos; 2. most of them felt their health was fairly good; 3. there was not much worry about their environment and they felt reasonably safe; 4. although they had government health insurance, it was difficult for them to get health care because of their language problems; 5. some of them felt lonely, others did not; 6. some felt seriously depressed – some wept during the interviews; 7. many said that their lack of English ability was a serious problem and that they could not watch television, take public transportation, use many commercial services, shop in many stores, speak to their neighbors, or get health care because of this problem; 8. many lived alone, their children having left the area to work elsewhere; 9. they greatly enjoyed going to the senior center to meet other Lao, but they could only go twice a week, when there was a program for them.

Step Six, Refining the Intuition: From this limited information, it looked as though the most important parts of the intuition were language problems and social isolation. The language problem interfered with their health care, nutrition, and exercise, and prevented them from having more social contacts, all of which were health challenges. Social isolation was a problem because of the geographic scattering of families, and the fact that the Lao community was spread out over a wide area as well. There were few things they could easily do to meet other Lao. Resources were the American welfare system, which gave them enough to live on, and the multicultural senior center, where they could meet other Lao.

Step Seven, Recommendations: It would have been better if the students had had more time to check on their conclusions. However, as an exercise, they thought about things that might be done to improve this situation. The most important need for the Lao was people to teach them English. The students discussed the possibility of asking American elderly volunteers to be organized to do this. A second need was for an expanded senior center program, and a third need was for culturally appropriate mental health services in the Lao language.

SUMMARY

The community-based approach to health and health care has many clear advantages, especially for communities with limited resources. In order to realize these advantages, health workers and health planners must make sure that they understand the social, cultural, economic, and environmental bases of health and illness in a given community. A knowledge of how local people view their own lives and health, and the strategies they use to get their needs met, is also important. Health anthropology provides a method for learning these things.

However, achieving health at the community level also means helping people to change their ways of thinking and acting. For this reason it is necessary to bring the local community itself into the search for improvements. This in turn requires a new way of looking at professionalism in the health sciences, a change from the role of the outside expert, to that of the student, advisor, and collaborator.

In some learning settings it is difficult for health professional students to understand and accept the model of professionalism that naturalistic research demands. Many have been trained to think of their profession in the old way – that of a distant, high status, knowledgeable expert bringing knowledge and care to people who need it. What is worse, some students have the belief that the conferring of a degree or certificate itself guarantees their ability to lead and to heal. This can lower their motivation for actually mastering the difficult skills and knowledge detailed in this book.

Students can learn the needed attitudes by observing and taking part in successful activities that are guided by these attitudes, far better than by studying abstract texts. Student-centered teaching creates a microculture in which the needed attitudes toward professionalism are modeled, practiced, and learned. It is a microculture that develops cooperative skills, curiosity, and self-confidence, and which students find energizing and enjoyable.

What I have outlined in this chapter is simply an example of that method, an example that was developed largely for American health science students, and adapted also for students from Thailand, South Africa, and Latin America. I am sure that there are many strategies and ideas that will work as well or better than these with other groups of students, and I invite you, teachers, to experiment with it, to adapt it to your unique situation and students.

CHAPTER THIRTEEN

Professionalism in Naturalistic Social Science

GUIDE TO THIS CHAPTER

In this chapter I would like to examine the current state of professionalism in social science research, and particularly, the issues of verification and objectivity that have been addressed throughout this book. I would like to explain how some naturalistic health researchers propose to address those issues, and then offer my own solution.

Most health professionals have spent years mastering knowledge based on the experimental sciences – biology, chemistry, physics, experimental psychology – and their clinical cousins such as pathology, anatomy, and pharmacology. These are the sciences, after all, that have led to nearly all of the important discoveries underlying modern diagnosis and treatment of disease. But this grounding in experimental science creates a problem for those who also want to master the naturalistic sciences – those social sciences that seek to understand things that cannot be dissected in a laboratory, such as communities, cultures, and personalities.

Throughout this book I have shown in various ways the difference between experimental and naturalistic validity, and I hope that you now understand that difference pretty well. Both methods have their advantages and disadvantages, and in this chapter I would like to address ways in which they can be used together for the ultimate goal of furthering research.

THE QUALITY OF NATURALISTIC RESEARCH

Many health scientists are already using naturalistic methods to try to solve problems that are known to have a social or psychological dimension (as I believe nearly all health problems do when we try to put their solutions into practice in human communities). But there seems to be little agreement or clarity about the quality of this work, even among those who do it. As a recent article in a leading medical journal put it,

"Qualitative methods are now widely used and increasingly accepted in health research, but quality in qualitative research remains a mystery to many health services researchers" (May & Pope, 2000, p. 320).

As the practical value of qualitative social research gains acceptance in various applied fields, more and more scholars are publishing their views on this issue of the quality of such research. It is easy to get confused by this profusion of views. And so, I will begin by summarizing the specific problems addressed by this body of work, and the main solutions that are offered. Then I will expand on what I think is the best solution – the previously mentioned criterion of *usefulness* as the special form of validity by which such knowledge should be judged.

POSITIVIST-FRIENDLY NATURALISTIC METHOD

As we have discussed throughout this book (particularly in Chapter Three), those who would work in the naturalistic method face the conceptual issues of *verification* and *objectivity*.

The *problem of verification*, you may recall, refers to the fact that the data of naturalistic studies cannot be verified in some of the ways that experimental data can be – for example, by repeating the experiment or one very similar. As a result, using the positivist canons of the experimental sciences, there may not be a clear way to choose among two or more naturalistic accounts that disagree with one another.

The *problem of objectivity* refers to the fact that since social research itself is an expression of cultural behavior, it cannot be said to represent objective reality any more than the human beliefs that it describes.

Several qualitative researchers have addressed the conceptual problems of verification and objectivity and have offered intelligent solutions. I will outline some of these solutions here, and then explain why I have reached a different one.

May and Pope (2000) are especially interested in the problem of verification, and they suggest that it can be solved by taking a *modified* positivist approach. Their stand is based on the claim that it is possible in comparing various approaches to the understanding of any research problem, to assess the *relative* objectivity and validity of each. Naturalistic research can achieve a level of quality equal or superior to quantitative methods, they believe, as long as the research process is:

1. *Transparent*: The researcher must explain clearly and in detail how the data of the study were collected, and how they were analyzed, in such a way that the reader can imagine the process and judge whether it makes sense.

2. *Convincing*: A potential user of a piece of research will presumably have some knowledge about the topic – either the group or the health issue that was studied, or both. This fund of inexact background knowledge gives the reader the ability to decide whether the research follows general observations and principles of deduction, or not.

3. *Thorough*: Ideally, the researchers should use an array of methods, and consider seriously any information that might call their findings into question, such as respondent skepticism, negative cases, and alternative explanations.

4. *Relevant*: Does the research actually address the problems that the reader is interested in? It is often tempting to use general data about a particular group or situation and try to interpret what it means in terms of the research question that the reader has in mind. But this is risky. The reader must be careful only to rely on studies that actually focus on the issue at hand. I will return to this problem shortly.

Henwood and Pidgeon (1993) take an almost identical position. For them, the goals of naturalistic research are somewhat different from those of positivistic studies, aiming as they do at useful understanding rather than certainty. However, the former can be accepted as valid to the extent that: (a) interpretations are supported by recorded data; (b) accounts are *reflexive* – meaning that the researcher seeks to account for the effect of the observation itself on the observed phenomena; (c) the results are *integrated at various levels of abstraction*, meaning that they make sense not just in the case under direct observation, but also in terms of other work on it and similar topics; (d) the results are well-documented; (e) attention is paid to what population(s) the observed data can be said to represent; (f) cases which do not fit the analysis are considered in the explanation; (g) respondents are asked to validate the results; and, (h) the results are persuasive, given what is known about the subject.

A different kind of positivist friendly solution is offered by the sociologist Martyn Hammersley (2001) and by Hammersley and Atkinson (1995). Here, the problem of objectivity is taken seriously and thoroughly discussed, but radical relativism (the notion that all facts are essentially social constructs) is finally rejected on two grounds. First, pushed to its logical conclusion, it leads to the position that there is no way at all to judge the objectivity of any account, and all accounts are therefore equally biased. This of course renders social science inquiry as a whole almost senseless. The second argument against antirealism is that it results in the politicization of social science. If research is a hopelessly subjective process, one might as well use it selectively to support one's *a priori* political constructions.

Therefore, although we cannot fully transcend the *as if* quality of our analyses, Hammersley and Atkinson maintain that we can move toward certainty about the real world in much the same way that May and Pope outline in their discussion of quality in qualitative research. Hammersley (2001, p. 108) calls this position *subtle realism* – the struggle to achieve *reasonable confidence* that something is objectively true, without making the leap of faith required by positivism that there is actually a knowable truth *out there*. Like May and Pope, Hammersley and Atkinson also find the criterion of relevance important in assessing the confidence level of naturalistic research. Thus, "...all knowledge [not just naturalistic knowledge] is based on assumptions and purposes, and is a human construction..." (Hammersley, 2001, p. 109), and "[G]iven that what is produced [by ethnographers] is, at best, only one of many possible valid accounts of the phenomena studied, it is a requirement that ethnographers make explicit the relevance on which their accounts are based" (*ibid.*, p. 110).

On the problem of validation (which he does not separate from the problem of objectivity), Hammersley again agrees that replication of naturalistic research is extremely difficult, if not impossible. However, he insists that such research can be seen as *more or less* valid to the extent that: (a) the analyses are plausible, given what is known about the topic; (b) the analyses are credible, given what is known about the researchers, the site, and the topic; (c) the raw data are also plausible and credible; and, (d) the findings are important, insofar as they address issues worthy of scientific reporting. These criteria are adequate for Hammersley, in the context of the basic rules of scientific inquiry with which we are all familiar, namely: (a) all findings are subject to assessment by the community of scholars; (b) researchers are always willing to change their assessment of a subject in the light of convincing evidence; and, (c) anyone who is willing to play by these rules may participate in the evaluation (Hammersley, 1998). In short, replicability of naturalistic findings is not necessary, as long as the community of scholars knowledgeable about the general subject area find them plausible, credible, and interesting.

USEFULNESS AS VALIDITY: A BETTER SOLUTION

These are interesting and intelligent attempts to solve the problems of verification and objectivity, but I am not completely satisfied with them. I do not think they help health scientists who are deeply committed to their own positivist view of reality to apply naturalistic methods wisely.

Objection No. 1: The Problem of Values

First, these positivist-friendly solutions have a serious logical flaw. They continue to refer to the search for durable, objective laws (agreement among observations, among observers or participants, among methods, among levels of analysis, and among scholars), while at the same time admitting that the logic of social analysis is not universal, and therefore acknowledging the moral, non-logical, importance of *interest or usefulness* in assessing the adequacy of research. I shall call this the *problem of values*.

There is a long and rich history in the philosophy of knowledge that supports exactly this idea of scientific truth, the tradition called *pragmatism* (Dewey, 1984), but these positivist-friendly theorists do not mention the pragmatist tradition. This is not the place for a thorough discussion of pragmatism; I need only note that it is a respected tradition in the philosophy of science, and simply holds that *the essential test of the validity of a scientific observation is its practical usefulness*. Throughout this book, I have explained how health scientists can use the pragmatist idea of usefulness to make clear to their positivist colleagues the value, and the *validity*, of naturalistic research.

Objection No. 2: The Problem of Shared Tradition

My second reason for challenging positivist-friendly solutions to the problem of verification is this: Such solutions require that the researcher, and the research user, have a professional sense of what is *reasonable* at all levels of observation and analysis. Having a professional sense of validity means that the makers and users of naturalistic research must have considerable experience in studying and using this kind of research, just as professional social scientists have, in order to get a feel for what makes sense. One must have participated in a community of scholars concerned with the kind of work one is trying to evaluate or accomplish. This requirement puts these positivist-friendly solutions out of the reach of most health professionals. Many nurses, public health workers, doctors, health science educators, and health policy makers recognize the potential benefits of qualitative studies, but are ill-at-ease performing or using such studies because they know they lack the experience that alone permits confident judgment of reasonability, according to the standards that social scientists themselves use. I shall call this the *problem of shared tradition*.

The idea of *usefulness as validity* solves the problem of values by admitting that the answer to any valid question in naturalistic science is a useful understanding of a practical problem. Since virtually no solution is useful unless it convinces others of its accuracy, of course the researcher must also understand what sorts of evidence are persuasive to his or her colleagues, and show how the research is supported by that kind of evidence.

In addition to solving the problem of values, the idea of usefulness as validity ends up offering considerable relief from the problem of shared tradition as well. Pragmatism recognizes clearly, and incorporates thoroughly, what positivist-friendly apologists for naturalistic social science try to smuggle in through a side door: that the way human beings ordinarily know most things and solve most problems is adequate for social science; and that this ordinary way of knowing is inseparable from our interests and intentions. Health scientists belong to professions (medicine, nursing, public health, and so on) that have well-developed traditions according to what is, and is not, useful: standard, experimental, and alternative ideas concerning the causal pathways of disease and healing, diagnostic methods, treatment standards, principles of care, health promotion techniques, professional ethics, teaching skills, and so on, make up the culture of practice in each professional community. These cultures of practice in turn structure the interests of health professionals that guide the selection of research problems, and the recognition of quality in research results. The principle of usefulness as the criterion of validity allows each professional to draw on knowledge of these traditions to make judgments about the value of research, as well as to persuade colleagues of that value.

Recognizing that it is usefulness itself that distinguishes knowledge from other perceptions, and understanding that the degree of usefulness is what separates more excellent from less excellent knowledge, add two more weapons to the arsenal of the naturalistic health science researcher.

First, they free us from the need to describe naturalistic science apologetically as a kind of watered-down certainty. Often enough, naturalistic studies are far more useful than quasi-experimental ones when applied to complex human problems, and their usefulness can make up for any lack of precision.

Second, they free us from the need to apologize for the application of our own values, or ethics, in the evaluation of scientific work. As long as we make our values clear (to ourselves as well as others) we can explain our support for a particular analysis in a way that makes sense to other scientists.

The chief objection to the inclusion of usefulness at the expense of universality as a criterion of scientific knowledge is that this opens science to the accusation of political bias. I am aware of two types of defense against this accusation. First, there is the long-standing argument that, given the intractability of the problem of objectivity, all social science is value-laden in any case, and it is better to recognize this fact at the start.

A good social researcher should state his or her values and aims as clearly as possible at the outset, and allow them to be included in any evaluation of the work (*Cf.* Gouldner, 1963; Hammersley, 1995, p. 16). The second is that in laying bare the assumptions and strategies of all stakeholders in a social situation, social science often has the effect of redistributing some of the knowledge-power that each stakeholder seeks to control, thereby supporting the widespread value of human equality. In the search for the most broadly useful understandings, the political stance of the social science researcher is often *anti-political*, that is, making people more conscious of, and thereby implicitly questioning, the status quo or the direction of existing processes of change.

ASSESSING COMMUNITY HEALTH BELIEFS

In order to clarify this argument, let us examine a single example of a common way health professionals and applied social scientists use naturalistic research to address real needs in communities (covered in Chapters 9, 10, and 11). Since public opinion can play a large role in mobilizing people to change their behavior or environment, many health agencies now recognize the benefits of assessing the subjective beliefs that community residents have about threats to their health, in addition to the so-called objective measures of ill health such as rates of hypertension or infectious disease. Naturalistic method, if done properly, is particularly suited to assessing such beliefs, because it is sensitive to the interactions of belief, behavior, and context. However, trained as most are in positivist methods, health professionals are plagued by several related problems in assessing community health beliefs.

They are inclined to begin by assuming that there is an objective set of health beliefs *out there,* and that their job is to measure this set objectively. In the process, they overlook the situated and negotiated nature of such health beliefs – the fact that the beliefs they are likely to elicit are the products of what Gubrium (1988, p. 13) calls *logics in use* – ideas adhering to discoverable principles of social action shared by the community, but profoundly affected by, among other things, the context of the research.

Such an accounting derives from a complex understanding of *what the logics are* that people are using to shape their responses – how they view the researchers and the research situation, why this makes sense in the local culture and experience, what kinds of actions might change this equation. The need to assess these things, in turn, in a way that rises to a level of scientific objectivity, in the absence of thorough professionalism in social research, can be deeply discouraging to even the most committed health professionals. They may turn away from naturalistic research in the face of such problems and simply revert to their professional habit of *managing* solutions without adequate knowledge of their impact. They may prefer the highly impractical but widely accepted approach of using positivist criteria of validity in the data collection, seeking not only to draw causal inferences and act on it locally, but also to generalize from it to a wider population, with almost certainly disappointing results.

The matter of local health beliefs is seen in a different light under a pragmatist approach. Here, it is legitimate for the health professionals to look at field research not as an attempt at objective assessment at all, but rather as a negotiation, in which the perceived interests and needs of community members, and those of the researchers, are clarified in search of a common understanding that will be as satisfactory as possible to as many participants as possible. Any such understanding must be based on the idea of action – what can be done, practically speaking, to improve the well-being of the community? Any such process will combine data collection, analysis, and the testing of conclusions through application. John Dewey was the chief architect of the idea of usefulness as validity. He wrote, "The quest for certainty by means of exact possession in mind of immutable reality is exchanged for search for security by means of active control of the changing course of events" (Dewey, 1984, p. 163).

It might be argued that the result of such a process will not be recognizable as social science at all; that it will amount to the ad hoc borrowing of techniques and vocabulary from naturalistic research in order to give an air of respectability to an otherwise informal and somewhat chaotic process. At first, and in some cases, this might be one useful way of looking at it. On the other side of the argument: (a) any health scientist who is interested can take a look at the philosophy of science and find that the idea of usefulness as validity holds a distinguished position there; and (b) using pragmatist epistemology to cut through the problems that deter health professionals from using naturalistic studies could open up a new partnership between experimental and naturalistic science. Such a viewpoint might clear the way for both kinds of scientists to use each other's findings more creatively. In the long run, this might lead to a convergence of the social and health sciences among the growing group of scholars and practitioners whose interests lie in both communities.

SUMMARY

The health professional who decides to incorporate naturalistic social research methods and findings in his or her work today adopts a potentially powerful tool for the development of more effective health interventions, at both the individual and community levels. At the same time, this decision involves the acceptance of a serious challenge – how to gain general recognition of one's naturalistic work within the professional cultures of one's colleagues. This chapter summarizes recent published thinking on this problem, and offers what I believe is an improvement – the clear and straightforward use of utility as the principle measure of scientific validity. This position – *pragmatism* – is a well-developed and well-respected one in the philosophy of science. The health scientist who is able to translate it into terms acceptable to the cultures of the health professions may well have found a way to incorporate within those cultures the distinctive power of naturalistic social science.

A Scoring System for Need Satisfaction Values

The *Theory of Needs* (Chapter Nine) proposes that individual life-styles and decision processes can be understood as strategies for meeting personal needs within the context of a culture and an environment. These personal strategies can be roughly understood by applying the theory analytically to ordinary ethnographic data.

To get a more thorough and complete idea of needs and satisfactions for individuals, and to compare settings or measure changes over time, it is helpful to have a standard scoring system for assessing how well or how poorly need satisfaction strategies seem to be working. This is such a scoring system. Researchers who wish to use the theory of needs to understand health-related behaviors are encouraged use it, adapting it to their own particular research problems and settings.

The following system is self-explanatory. For each of the five needs, it lists the criteria to be used to classify any situation, behavior, or belief as either a potential source of satisfaction of that need, or a potential deprivation with respect to that need. Complex behaviors might fulfill several criteria of one need, or of several needs. In some cases, behaviors might function as satisfactions in one respect, and threats in another respect. All these values should be scored for every behavior of interest.

In many cases, *the perception of the research subject(s) and that of the researcher may differ with respect to the value of a behavior.* Thus, each behavior should be scored twice: once from the perspective of the researcher, and again from the perspective of the subject(s), to the extent that perspective is known.

I. SECURITY

A. Satisfaction

Might this situation, behavior, or way of thinking:

- contribute to (strengthen), now or in the future, resources necessary for life, such as money, shelter, food, health or health care, freedom from harm, warmth, and so forth? One's job, family, work and self-care skills, health, perceived environmental resources, friendships, reputation, beliefs in divine help or magic, stocks of useful goods or money, all might provide satisfactions;
- make the future more predictable, reducing uncertainty about essential things, such as where and how one will live, or what will happen if current sources of security are threatened? Beliefs and practices concerning life after death are included here;
- strengthen social relationships that contribute to either point one or two, above?

B. Deprivation

Might this situation, behavior, or way of thinking:

- threaten (weaken) sources of security such as health, income, or supportive aspects of the environment? Technological change, insecurity of employment or of profit from work, physical or mental function loss due to illness or aging, or the instability of supportive social relationships are common examples;
- cause one's knowledge or skills to become useless? Changes that replace familiar work, familiar surroundings, and familiar social relations with unfamiliar ones might lower one's sense of security. Migration or change of residence often has this effect.

II. RESPECT

A. Satisfaction

Might this situation, behavior, or way of thinking:

- maintain or increase social status, now or in the future? Success in finances, competitive activities or games, love and marriage, or any socially recognized achievement (including offspring) may qualify, as well as acquisition of new goods, skills, or valued personal traits (beauty, wisdom), and contributions to the public good such as donations of money or work, exercising leadership, or confronting a public menace. Entry into a high status group or position might be important;

- reduce or remove a social stigma, such as overcoming a disability, a stigmatized condition such as poverty, a dishonorable profession, or a bad reputation?
- affirm and support one's sense of dignity and personal integrity, including cherished beliefs and behaviors? Approval of acts and ideas that one identifies as one's own is an important satisfaction of respect needs;
- increase one's power to require respectful or compliant behavior from others in the absence of genuine respect? Aggressive or dominating behavior belongs here.

B. Deprivation

Might this situation, behavior, or way of thinking:

- threaten a loss of social status or prestige, or block an expected increase in status? Included here are failure to perform socially approved functions, association with a stigmatized person or condition such as poverty or disease, loss of abilities needed to achieve respect, loss of a valuable title or asset, loss of respected personal qualities such as beauty or strength, and dependency on others. Note that social status is *relative*; an increase in the difference of status that leaves a person relatively lower on the social scale is perceived as a deprivation. Chronic illness, sensory loss, loss of job or income, and divorce are common deprivations of respect;
- interrupt relationships with those who appreciate one's status? Extended travel or migration away from family and community, or the illness, migration, disappearance or death of the members of one's family or community are frequent causes;
- show contempt or indifference toward ideas, behaviors, abilities, possessions, and people that are associated with self-respect? Especially on the part of powerful or high status people or agencies, failure to acknowledge the value of things that make us feel worthy.

III. LOVE

A. Satisfaction

Might this situation, behavior, or way of thinking:

- increase or maintain the amount of contact with intimate others? Examples are marriage or living together, working or playing together with friends or family, taking care of or doing favors for loved ones, or depending on them for help or care. Being ill can often supply satisfaction of the need for love. Note: love is usually reciprocal – being loved by those for whom the individual has little feeling is of little value;

- increase one's feelings of being known and appreciated by others? Examples are the formation or deepening of loving relationships with people or pets, the birth of children or grandchildren, and sexual intimacy;

- increase one's sense of security that a loving relationship will continue in the future? Since love relationships can be highly unstable and this instability can be extremely painful, most people will exert great effort to form more stable relationships, and protect those they have against disruption. Membership in an organization or gang often has this function. Jealousy is an expression of this need.

B. Deprivation

Might this situation, behavior, or way of thinking:

- decrease contact with loved others? Any decrease in the frequency and duration of contact with loved others can be felt as a deprivation. Again, migration or change of residence of the self or loved others, or the commitment of their time to other relationships belongs here;

- decrease the depth or intensity of shared feelings? This includes loss of the affection of those whose love is expected, increased competition with others, or decreased ability of either partner to express love or engage in activities that strengthen love;

- threaten the well-being of a significant other? People will often work to protect those who satisfy their need for love.

IV. MEANING

A. Satisfaction

Might this situation, behavior, or way of thinking:

- affirm one's beliefs and values? Contact with others who share one's beliefs and values, especially in situations where those beliefs are clearly expressed, such as rituals, or group work that serves a valued cause. People will often strive to preserve and strengthen their culture, religion, and political alliances. Events that bear out one's predictions of the future – good or bad – add value to one's beliefs;

- preserve or increase experience of the familiar? Familiar persons, places, activities, and events – or even those that resemble the familiar – carry powerful meaning, because they are associated with the individual's sense of what is normal. This can even be true of stressful experiences and relationships;
- reduce one's sense of uncertainty or confusion? The feeling of not knowing what to do is often extremely stressful. Following a fixed routine and avoiding situations and topics that are poorly understood serves this need. Another important strategy is the psychological habit of denial – simply refusing to admit the reality of things that do not fit one's knowledge base.

B. Deprivation

Might this situation, behavior, or way of thinking:

- undermine or contradict one's beliefs and values? Being presented, especially by a powerful person or agency, with views or actions that place our own in doubt can raise confusion and uncertainty. Especially difficult is evidence that others do not understand or accept our view of ourselves – of who we are. This is a source of much class and cultural conflict;
- reduce the experience of familiarity? Extensive change in one's surroundings, especially when sudden, but even when gradual, can reduce one's sense of meaning. The changes associated with migration, culture change, and the aging of one's body are usually deprivations. Even positive changes such as increased prosperity or improved environment can bring on feelings of meaninglessness;
- block access to one's goals, or render one's need satisfaction strategies useless? The discovery that a valued future is impossible can produce a crisis in meaning, in which one's beliefs and assumptions suddenly seem false or valueless. This is a common cause of depression.

V. STIMULATION

A. Satisfaction

Might this situation, behavior, or way of thinking:

- preserve or improve one's access to a variety of non-offensive experiences? (I use the term *non-offensive* rather than *pleasant*, because stimulation is sought for its own sake, and need not be consciously felt as pleasant.) Does it protect or enlarge one's amount and variety of entertainment, food or drink, art or music, conversation, sports, travel, sex, hobby activity, danger, central nervous system arousal (drugs, meditation, trance), interesting work, or simply novel situations? Note the importance for health – many kinds of desired stimulation involve major health risks;

- preserve or promote one's physical or mental ability to pursue stimulation? Strength and stamina, sensory or mental clarity, physical attractiveness, knowledge, energy, and skills – especially social skills – are needed to pursue many kinds of stimulation. Health-promoting behavior and the pursuit of education and training often have this goal.

B. Deprivation

Might this situation, behavior, or way of thinking:

- block or reduce access to stimulating experience? Common deprivations include lack of resources, poor health, lack of energy, lack of knowledge or skills, social isolation, stigma or low status, loss of close relationships, lack of time free from routine activities, and preoccupation with threats to other needs. For the elderly, loss of relationships, health, strength, sensory clarity, and mental ability often lead to severe deprivation of stimulation. This is another important health problem. Deprivation of stimulation is related to decline in both cognitive and physical functioning, and to an increase in depression.

References

Anderson, E. (1990). *Street wise: Race, class, and change in an urban community.* Chicago: University of Chicago Press.

Becker, H. (2001). The epistemology of qualitative research. In R. Emerson (Ed.), *Contemporary field research: Perspectives and formulations* (2nd ed., pp. 317–330). Prospect Heights, IL: Waveland.

Benitez, D. (1992). *Cooperativas de cristal.* Quetzaltenango, Guatemala: Talleres Litomarca.

Berger, P., & Luckman, T. (1967). *The social construction of reality.* Hammondsworth, UK: Penguin.

Bourgois, P. (1995). *In search of respect.* Cambridge, UK: Cambridge University Press.

Cochran, M. (2002). Deweyan pragmatism and post-positivist social science in IR. *Millenium: Journal of International Studies, 31*(3), 525–548.

Couto, R. (1991). *Ain't gonna let nobody turn me round.* Philadelphia: Temple University Press.

De Grazia, S. (1949). *The political community.* Chicago: University of Chicago Press.

Dewey, J. (1984). The quest for certainty. In J. A. Boydson (Ed.), *John Dewey: The later works, 1925–1953: 1929,* Vol. 4. Carbondale, IL: Southern Illinois University Press.

Durkheim, E. (1950). *The rules of sociological method.* G. E. Catlin (Ed.), S. Solray & J. Mueller (Trans.). New York: Free Press of Glencoe.

Durkheim, E. (1951). *Suicide.* G. Simpson (Ed.), A. Spaulding & G. Simpson (Trans.). New York: Free Press of Glencoe.

Frankl, V. (1959). *Man's search for meaning.* New York: Touchstone.

Geertz, C. (1972). Deep play: Notes on the Balinese cockfight. *Daedalus, 101,* 1–37.

Glazer, B., & Strauss, A. (1967). *The discovery of grounded theory.* Chicago: Aldine.

Gouldner, A. (1963). Anti-Minotaur: The myth of a value-free sociology. In M. Stein & A. Vidich (Eds.), *Sociology on trial* (pp. 35–52). Englewood Cliffs, NJ: Prentice-Hall.

Gubrium, J. (1988). *Analyzing field reality*. London: Sage.

Habermas, J. (1978). *Knowledge and human interests*. London: Heineman Educational.

Hammersley, M. (1998). *Reading ethnographic research: A critical guide*. London: Longman.

Hammersley, M. (2001). Ethnography and realism. In R. Emerson (Ed.), *Contemporary field research: Perspectives and formulations* (2nd ed., pp. 102–111). Prospect Heights, IL: Waveland.

Hammersley, M., & Atkinson, P. (1995). *Ethnography: Principles in practice* (2nd ed.). London: Routledge.

Henwood, K., & Pidgeon, N. (1993). Qualitative research and psychological theorizing. In Hammersley M. (Ed.), *Social research: Philosophy, politics, and practice* (pp. 14–32). London: Sage.

Higginbotham, M., Freeman, S., Heading, G., & Saul, A. (2001). Cultural construction of risk: Heart disease in the New South Wales Coalfields, Australia. In N. Higginbotham, R. Briceño-León, & N. Johnson (Eds.), *Applying health social sciences: Best practice in the developing world* (pp. 38–65). London: Zed.

Ingham, J. (1986). *Mary, Michael, and Lucifer: Folk Catholicism in Central Mexico*. Austin: University of Texas Press.

James, W. (1948). The Sentiment of rationality. In A. Castell (Ed.), *Essays in Pragmatism by William James* (pp. 3–36). New York: Hafner.

Katz, M. (1989). *The undeserving poor*. New York: Pantheon.

Kiefer, C. (1979). Loneliness in Japan. In R. Audy, R. Cohen, & J. Hartog (Eds.), *The anatomy of loneliness* (pp. 425–450). New York: International Universities Press.

Kiefer, C. (1988). *The mantle of maturity*. Albany, NY: SUNY Press.

Kiefer, C. (2000). *Health work with the poor*. New Brunswick, NJ: Rutgers University Press.

Kotlowitz, A. (1991). *There are no children here*. New York: Anchor Books.

Kozol, J. (1995). *Amazing grace: The lives of children and the conscience of a nation*. New York: Crown Books.

Lewis, O. (1951). *Life in a Mexican village: Tepoztlán restudied*. Urbana, IL: University of Illinois Press.

Lofland, J. (1967). Notes on naturalism. *Kansas Journal of Sociology, 3*(2), 45–61.

May, N., & Pope, C. (2000). Assessing quality in qualitative research. *British Medical Journal, 320*, 50–52.

Mills, C. W. (1959). *The sociological imagination*. Oxford: Oxford University Press.

Ramphele, M. (1997). Political widowhood in South Africa: The embodiment of ambiguity. In A. Kleinman, V. Das, & M. Lock (Eds.), *Social suffering* (pp. 99–118). Berkeley: University of California Press.

Redfield, R. (1930). *Tepoztlán, A Mexican village: A study of folk life*. Chicago: University of Chicago Press.

Rowe, M. (1999). *Crossing the border: Encounters between homeless people and outreach workers*. Berkeley: University of California Press.

Skinner, J. (2003, November). *Community protective factors and psychosocial resiliency: Community organizing in a Colombian war zone*. Presentation given at the annual meeting of American Public Health Association, San Francisco.

Stringer, E. (1996). *Action research: A handbook for practitioners*. Thousand Oaks, CA: Sage Publications.

Tarlo, E. (2003). *Unsettling memories: Narratives of the emergency in Delhi*. Berkeley: University of California Press.

Ten Have, P. (2004). *Understanding qualitative research and ethnomethodology*. London: Sage.

Tsing, A. (1993). *In the realm of the diamond queen: Marginality in an out-of-the-way place*. Princeton: Princeton University Press.

Weber, M. (1962). *Basic concepts in sociology*. New York: Philosophical Library.

WHO/UNICEF. (1978). *Non-governmental organizations and primary health care: A position paper/sponsored by WHO/UNICEF*. Halifax, Canada: World Federation of Public Health Organizations.

Zborowski, M., & Herzog, E. (1962). *Life is with people: The culture of the shtetl*. New York: Schoken Books.

Index

academic programs. *See also*
  training programs
in social medicine, 158
academic research, action
  anthropology *vs.*,
  197
accommodation process, in
  human patterning, 165–166
action anthropology, 92, 115,
  180, 202
  academic research *vs.*, 197
  adaptability and, 211
  challenges faced by, 201
  change facilitation in,
  205–211
  communication in, 210
  community empowerment
  and, 201–203
  inclusion in, 210
  intellectual function of,
  211–212
  leadership and, 197
  limitations in, 203
  moral dimension of, 200
  naturalistic knowledge and,
  197
  participation in, 210
  process of, 203–211

relationships in, 209–210
  usefulness of, 212
Action Research (Stringer), 209
active participation, classroom
  strategy of, 224–225
activist
  researcher *vs.*, 211
  roles of, 211
adaptation
  by action anthropologist, 211
  cultural patterns and, 166
  pattern disruption in, 174
adolescents, 15
aesthetics, defined, 24
African Americans, health care
  system and, 15, 16
age, 15, 41
alcoholism
  community meaning of, 74–75
  understanding process about,
  74–75
Anderson, Elijah, 185, 186
annotation aid programs, 147
anomie and hopelessness,
  180–182
  causes of, 184
  Durkheim on, 182, 183,
  188–189, 190

cases
  collection of, 74
  comparison of, 73, 121,
    157
  in positivist research, 61
change
  effect of context, 167
  non-health needs impact by,
    175
  from outside, 179–180
  resistance to, 179
  Theory of Hope impact on,
    180
change agents, in communities,
    197
CHP. See Community Health
    Practice
civic pride, 187
classification questions, in data
    analysis, 137
classification trees, organization
    charts, in anthropological
    writing, 140
classroom strategy, 222–226
  of active participation,
    224–225
  brainstorming as, 223
  debate as, 223–224
  of films, videos, guest
    speakers, 225
  of food, 225–226
  game learning as, 223
  of humor, 222–223
  for larger classes, 226–227
  role playing as, 224
  student facilitators and, 225
  team problem solving as, 224
clients, researchers and, 28, 29
closed-ended interviews, 123
Cochran, Molly, 47

coding raw data, 147. See also
    content coding
COIL. See Community Outlook
    Improvement
communication, 205–206
  in action anthropology, 210
communities
  anthropological researcher
    and, 108
  change agents in, 197
  in CHP, 159
  definition of, 159
  health beliefs of, 243–244
  health problems of, 125
  hope in, 181–182
  outside change for, 179–180
  outsider liaisons and, 202–203
  outsider treatment of, 192
  power, influence in, 204
  recent major problem history
    in, 204
  resources of, 204
  self-worth and, 164–165
  self-awareness development
    in, 201–202
  self-healing, 187–188
  self-wounding, 173, 185–186
  shared characteristics of, 159
  social capital of, 186
  social change in, 212
  stakeholders in, 204
  as unique pattern, 113
community action, sustaining,
    211
community behavior, change of,
    179
community change
  alternative theory of, 190–191
  intuition about, 191–192
  theory impact on, 191–194

uniqueness, of culture, 5, 59–60
universe, basic laws of, 23
unobtrusive measures, 130–131
urban poor, Marxism impact on, 187
urge to know, 36
usefulness, 71, 238
  of action anthropology, 212
  of anthropological research, 198
  in anthropological writing, 152–153
  of laboratory sciences, 32
  in naturalistic theory, 36, 48, 189, 212
  as reliability, 240–243
  of research answers, 77–78
  of truth, 152
  as validity, 240–243

validity and reliability. *See also*
  of interviews, 125
  in laboratory sciences, 23

  in positivism, 26
  positivist *vs.* naturalistic, 47
  in process, 47
  usefulness as, 240–243
values, 93–96. *See also* Problem of Values
  in anthropological research, 79
verification. *See also* Problem of Verification
  of naturalistic social science, 45
  in social science research, 237
victimization, norms impact by, 184
violence 14, 75
visualization, hope and, 181

Weber, Max, 35
Wittgenstein, Ludwig, 125

Zborowsky, Mark, 185